Pain: Causes, Concerns and Consequences

Edited By:

Puneetpal Singh
&
Monica Singh
Human Genetics Punjabi University
Patiala
India

Bentham Science Publishers Ltd.
Executive Suite Y - 2
PO Box 7917, Saif Zone
Sharjah, U.A.E.
Email: subscriptions@benthamscience.org

BENTHAM
SCIENCE

CONTENTS

PREFACE

The present book is about pain, a vital part but an unwelcome guest in the corridors of human health. If we count the toll of human sufferings, the pain is the forefront perpetrator. It is metastasizing and has tethered directly or indirectly to almost every disease or morbid condition. Its realisation is different by anaesthesiologist on pre-operative condition, neurologist on migraine or headache, rheumatologist on arthritis and oncologist on cancer, however, complex and distinctive appraisals are proclaimed by different patients.

Scientist have exposed constellation of factors and started hunting down all those culprits which contribute but are still absconding from the scene of pain. The physiological, biochemical and genetic role in human pain has been delved, discussed and disseminated in clinical literature but many concerns are still to be unravelled.

This compendium, "Pain: Causes, Concerns and Consequences" is aimed to assimilate and harness scholastic knowledge from the scientists and researchers of high repute, who have been working in this domain of pain research. This treatise has positively brought state of the art knowledge in relation to prognosis and prophylactic measures of pain, which we surmise to be a valuable volume.

In the first chapter Dr. David shares his experiences of understanding pain as a clinician. He trudges along his memory lane and discusses the interdependence of clinician and researcher in the search of indepth perception of explained and unexplained pain. His professional journey as a special orthodontist proffers a novel way of tackling pain by employing not only classical but psychological ways and means.

Dr. Bai Chuang Shyu discussed that central post -stroke pain (CPSP) involves three hypotheses: central disinhibition, central imbalance and central sensitisation, which do not conflict with each other.

He puts forth that, although, neural substrates of CPSP are diverse, but cortical pain matrix (contra lateral somatosensory cortex, bilateral mid and posterior insula, interior insula and posterior cingulate cortex) regulates pain processing in CPSP. He concludes that [^{14}C] iodoantipyrine (IAP) data from the animal model of CPSP with lesions of ventrobasal complex of right thalamus indicate that during pain, significantly higher activation occurs in the medial prefrontal cortex (mPFC), interior cingulate cortex, thalamus, hypothalamus, amygdala and periaqueductal gray (PAG). He proposes that for, CPSP this novel idea of checking [^{14}C] IAP may be used for pharmacological and non- pharmacological interventions of CPSP.

Third chapter emphasises the psychological issues in cardiac and non-cardiac chest pain. In emergency departments and intensive cardiac care units (ICCU), the most common symptoms of these patients are psychological stress, fear and anxiety. If remain unaddressed, these symptoms may lead to worst outcomes with severe ramifications. Psychotherapy especially cognitive and behavioural interventions can substantially lower the pain developed as a consequence of psychological distress.

Fourth chapter presents the facts and figures of several genes that participate in different phases of pain. Pain being a complex manifestation is perceived, processed and promulgated first and foremost through genetic endowment of the individual whereas, physiology, psychology, sociology and environment, later appear on the scene. It is acknowledged in this chapter that the idea of personal medicine for managing pain, based on the genetic profiling of the individual is possible in near future.

Dr Przekop writes about the causes and concerns of chronic non-cancer pain (CNCP) especially when coexisted with substance use disorder (SUD). He professes that, in formulating the treatment plan for CNCP and SUD the concomitant factors of one's psychology, sociology and physiology should be taken care of, so that the patient becomes an active participant in the treatment of his or her chronic pain.

Fifth chapter emerges out from a query that whether microRNAs (miRNAs) play role in pain pathophysiology and targeting them can be useful in managing pain. The chapter diligently explores the role and relevance of miRNAs in anti-nociceptive therapeutics. Apropos to the query, the chapter reveals that understanding the miRNA expression profile in almost every component of somatosensory system from peripheral neurons to higher central system, plays promising role in modulation of pain perception.

Dr Muthuraman investigates the analgesic potential of 7-hydoxy-4-methyl-coumarin (HMC) in acrylamide induced pain in rats. By conducting acrylamide induced nociceptive pain sensation and biochemical estimation, he documents that pre-treatment of rats with HMC and cyclosporine; ameliorate the acrylamide induced changes in biochemical and behavioural parameters in dose dependent manner.

He suggests that this ameliorative effect of HMC is because of its antioxidant, anti-lipid peroxidative, calcium ion regulatory and mitochondrial permeability transition pore inhibitory action.

We are deeply indebted to Ms. ShalluKhullar for her extended help in style editing of the book. We extend our heartfelt gratitude to Mrs. Humaira Hashmi, Editor In-charge, eBook department and Editorial Manager Publications, Ms. Hira Aftab, Incharge Publications, Ms. Maria Baig, Manager Publications and especially Mr.MahmoodAlam, Director Publications,

Bentham Science publishers for their kind support, encouragement and help.

Dr. Puneetpal Singh
Department of Human Genetics
Punjabi University, Patiala, India
Dr. Monica Singh
Department of Human Genetics
Punjabi University, Patiala, India

List of Contributors

Andrew Chih Wei Huang	Department of Psychology, Fo Guang University, Yilan, Taiwan, Republic of China
Arunachalam Muthuraman	Neuropharmacology Division, Department of Pharmacology and Toxicology, Akal College of Pharmacy & technical Education, Mastuana Sahib, Sangrur 148002, Punjab, India
Bai Chuang Shyu	Institute of Biomedical Sciences, Academia Sinica, Taipei, Taiwan, Republic of China
David S. Basser	53 Bennetts Road Mountain River, Tasmania 7109, Australia
Harjot Dhillon	Department of Human Genetics, Punjabi University, Patiala, India
Hsiang-Chin Lu	Institute of Biomedical Sciences, Academia Sinica, Taipei, Taiwan, India
Jaspreet Kaur	Neuropharmacology Division, Department of Pharmacology and Toxicology, Akal College of Pharmacy & technical Education, Mastuana Sahib, Sangrur 148002, Punjab, India
Masoumali Masoumi	Professor of Cardiac Surgery, Bistoon Hospital, Kermanshah, Iran
Mozhgan Saeid	Cardiac Rehabilitation Center, Imam Ali Hospital, Kermanshah University of Medical Sciences, Kermanshah, Iran
Muthusaamy Ramesh	Neuropharmacology Division, Department of Pharmacology and Toxicology, Akal College of Pharmacy & technical Education, Mastuana Sahib, Sangrur 148002, Punjab, India
Peter Przekop	Betty Ford Center, Rancho Mirage, CA 92270, USA, Departments of Pediatrics, Neurology, and Psychiatry. Loma Linda University School of Medicine, Loma Linda, CA 92350, USA
Puneetpal Singh	Department of Human Genetics, Punjabi University, Patiala, India
Saeid Komasi	Cardiac Rehabilitation Center, Imam Ali Hospital, Kermanshah University of Medical Sciences, Kermanshah, Iran
Yogita K. Adlakha	Cellular and Molecular Neuroscience, National Brain Research Centre, Manesar-122051, India

Pain: Causes, Concerns and Consequences

DEDICATION

Our Parents and Dear Son Bunny

CHAPTER 1

Pain: A Clinician's Journey

David S. Basser*

22 High Street New Norfolk, Tasmania 7140, Australia

Abstract: Pain is a percept: it is an unpleasant sensory and emotional experience, a product of the brain's abstraction that might be considered an activity mediated event: the activity being the message and pain the messenger warning of imminent or actual injury or imbalance yet to be avoided or resolved. There are no 'painful stimuli' that is stimuli that invariably elicit the perception of pain in all individuals and it is this highly individual and subjective nature of pain that makes it difficult to define and to treat clinically. The key to understanding and therefore appropriate treatment is in deciphering the message. Recognising and respecting the interdependence of both the clinician and researcher in the search for deeper discernment proffers the potential for synergistic evolution in understanding and treatment with the promise of bringing relief to many sufferers of both explained and unexplained pain.

Keywords: Allodynia, Central sensitisation, Chronic pain, Clinical application, Clinical experience, Global syndrome, Idiopathic pain, Neural activity, Neuroplasticity, Occlusion, Orofacial pain, Pain, Patient centred, Persistent pain, Precision medicine, Psychoneuroimmunology, Psychosocial, TMD.

INTRODUCTION

Pain and suffering are integral to the transformative journey that is life. In humans pain may be initiated at the physical, psychosocial and/or spiritual level(s) and experienced at any one or combination of these levels.

* **Corresponding author David S. Basser:** Specialist Dentist, 22 High Street New Norfolk, Tasmania 7140, Australia; Email: dbasser@ozonline.com.au.

Puneetpal Singh (Ed.)

PART 1

Pain: a Clinician's journey

There is an abundance of information in the scientific literature, the relevance of which is often beyond the scope of understanding of the general clinician. Likewise much of the clinical experience and effectiveness of the clinical generations is not part of the scope of conception of the general scientific researcher. In an age, demanding evidence based biomedicine, it would seem prudent to afford equal respect to the expertise developed in both clinical and research areas and acknowledge, through action, their interdependence to affect mutual synergistic evolution. This then may re-establish the balance, as called for by Besedovsky and Del Rey [1], between deduction and induction, analysis and synthesis (the essence of science) in biomedicine. Benjamin Moffett [2], Professor of Orthodontics at the University of Washington, School of Dentistry, afforded much respect in 1978: he stated, "As a professional scientist working in dentistry for the past 25 years, I have been impressed by the progress, which clinicians make with time in solving their patient's problems. These advances are often accomplished empirically without prior benefit of needed biological data from non-clinicians. Such gains are hard fought victories and are slowly recognized both within and outside the profession for several reasons. They are usually founded on individual clinical experience – a process that is not easily evaluated by others. Also the biological significance of these clinical advances is often obscured by the emphasis which clinicians naturally place on clinical procedures. But for those who are willing to learn from the trials and errors of others, the resulting insights are rewarding ... Because I am not a clinician ... you may be wondering why I opened the paper with a purely clinical observation. My reason is that when asked for a biological appraisal ... I ask the clinician in turn 'Does it work at the clinical level?' Whether a procedure or concept succeeds clinically is a big factor in determining its biological validity ... my question should (then) be (not if but) 'Why does it work?'"

I come to an understanding of pain having directly experienced two generations of clinical expertise in resolving patient's acute and chronic orofacial pain, the latter usually being classified as "idiopathic" or, to quote Woolf [3], "unexplained clinical pain".

In 2002, I embarked on a scientist's path in the quest for an explanation of the "unexplained". In November 2004, whilst completing a library based research paper in fulfilment of a unit for the formal neuroscience degree in which I was enrolled, I happened upon a theoretical explanation; the result of a distillation of the scientific literature combined with the experience and deliberations of two generations of clinicians. In line with Moffett's commentary, the paper (in a slightly updated form) did not find publication until 2012 [4]. Here, I present an updated theoretical understanding of pain based upon the clinical and scientific experience of the intervening years.

Pain; A Theoretical and Applied, Integrative Clinical and Research Understanding

"The sensation we call pain – pricking, burning, aching, stinging, and soreness - ... is a submodality of somatic sensation like touch, pressure and position sense and serves an important protective function. It warns of injury that should be avoided or treated. Pain is a percept: it is an unpleasant sensory and emotional experience... a product of the brain's abstraction and elaboration of sensory input... there are no 'painful stimuli' – stimuli that invariably elicit the perception of pain in all individuals"... thus... "The highly individual and subjective nature of pain is one of the factors that make it difficult to define and to treat clinically" [5].

All pain, might be considered an activity mediated event: the activity being the message and pain the messenger warning of imminent or actual injury or imbalance yet to be avoided or resolved. The key to understanding, and therefore appropriate treatment, will be in deciphering the message. When attempting to do so, it should be remembered that pain is not a site specific phenomenon, but a perception of activity mediated by the neural pain matrix which comprises a vast interrelated network of peripheral and central neural components acting as a functional unit [4].

From a neuroscientific perspective there are two aspects to consider, the pain threshold and the level of activity. The pain threshold might be thought of as an activity switch, the parameters of which are unique to each individual, being determined by a combination of their genetic disposition and total history of their physical and psychosocial activity (ie. experience). Pain is perceived when the net level of activity exceeds the pain threshold turning the switch on, and it is resolved when the net level drops below the threshold thereby turning the switch off. The net activity level required in any individual may vary from moment to moment, day to day, week to week, month to month, and year to year; this variation being an example of the neuroscientific phenomenon of *NERUOPLASTICITY.*

Pain (the messenger) is non-specific, it merely indicates that activity (the message) is being generated by physical and/or psychosocial phenomena at a level above the individual's pain threshold, and it is by systematically following clinical diagnostic protocols that the sources of the activity and their relative contribution might be revealed, as well as the status and underlying determinants of the pain threshold. Simply put, the clinician seeks to know *what is generating the activity, and what is the relative importance of the pain threshold?*

In dental practice, when the source of the message (activity) is a pathology associated with dentoalveolar structures then the diagnosis will often become obvious with conventional history and clinical diagnostic procedures that are based on anatomo-physiological concepts. An example of this is, when a patient provides a history of toothache radiating to the ear which commonly indicates pathology associated with the mandibular (lower jaw) structures. Another is when a tooth that is tender to percussion (tapping with a hand-instrument) and provides a negative result to pulp testing exhibits a periapical radiolucency indicative of pulpal necrosis (dental abscess). Where the cause of activity generation becomes less obvious and the pain is more persistent, especially in cases classified as examples of any of the chronic idiopathic orofacial pain entities, additional history and diagnostic procedures based on the neuroscientific principles and understandings associated with total body activity, both current and historical, provide the potential for deeper discernment and appropriate treatment [4]. In these patients, uncovering the circumstances around which the pain first appeared and the history of subsequent episodes will often provide insight into the relative contribution of physical and psychosocial factors to neural system sensitization which appears to play a central role in both acute and chronic pain perception [4,

6]. Central sensitization, the prolonged but reversible increase in the excitability and synaptic efficacy of neurons in central nociceptive pathways, is responsible for many of the accompanying temporal, spatial, and threshold changes in pain sensibility. These activity-dependent changes are triggered and maintained by dynamic nociceptor inputs and shift the sensitivity of the pain system, so that normally innocuous inputs can activate it (this phenomenon is known as *allodynia*) and the perceptual responses to noxious inputs are exaggerated, prolonged and wide spread; this understanding is the culmination of 25 years of research [3, 6]. In 2004, after two generations and 50 years of clinical practice, the theoretical explanation of chronic pain can be expressed as the equation:

Persistent (Chronic) Pain [PP] = Neural Activity [NA] cs + Neural Activity [NA] critical i.e. PP = NA (cs) + NA (critical)

Where NA (cs) is the neural activity required to induce central sensitization, and NA (critical) is the minimum level (or greater) of ongoing neural activity required to induce/maintain the pain and below which the pain resolves [4].

Within both the clinical and research communities, idiopathic pain entities continue to be seen as abnormal and therefore considered as pathology to be treated. It is thought that the healing function of the nervous system has gone "awry" when there is no noxious stimulus nor inflammation or damage to the nervous system [7]; this occurs in conditions like fibromyalgia, chronic tension-type headache, irritable bowel syndrome, chronic fatigue, lower back pain, major depression, panic attacks and post-traumatic stress disorder. These together with the idiopathic orofacial pain entities exhibit a co-morbidity leading to the conclusion that these conditions share a common aetiology [8]. Woolf [3] has suggested that these so called different syndromes may actually be different manifestations of central sensitization syndrome (with the inference/assumption of central sensitization being defective). A corollary to this might be that chronic pain can be considered as a manifestation of central sensitization, rather than focusing on a site-symptomatological description. The explanation/diagnosis of which would provide a clearer picture by uncovering the underlying associated neuroscientific phenomena.

This is the approach, I took in 2004 whilst seeking an explanation for the effective resolution of the chronic idiopathic head and neck pains (including those which would be classified as temporomandibular disorders [TMD]) achieved in my father's and my clinical practice following the considered and meticulous occlusal adjustment (selective shaving) of the teeth in numerous patients over more than 35 years. Two key questions were posed: 1) *What if chronic idiopathic orofacial pain was viewed from a neuroscientific perspective as part of a global syndrome rather than a site-symptom perspective*? 2) *What if it was assumed that rather than serving no useful purpose chronic idiopathic orofacial pain served a useful purpose*? [4].

Based on the neuroscientific understanding derived from my explorations I now provide a clinician's explanation (in words used for greater general understanding) for the existence of persistent pain. Initially the nervous system is "bruised" by trauma inducing neural overload and this "bruising" is maintained (prodded) by the total neural activity of the system irrespective of its origin; that is, the ongoing activity may be related to the initiating trauma or completely independent of it. The persistent pain, being the normal protective healing function of the nervous system, continues its warning. The key to pain relief is the reduction of the net ongoing activity of the nervous system to lower the pain threshold and ideally to a level where the "bruising" can resolve.

In my practice, clinical examples of trauma experienced by patients around the time when their pain first appeared, has varied from the physical disruption of a car accident to the psychological anguish of the death of a child. The working clinical hypothesis for the two examples mentioned was that both traumas produced sufficient neural activity to induce central sensitization and by reducing the net level of neural activity of the system, irrespective of source, would allow the normal mechanisms of neuroplasticity to restore the system towards its pre-trauma state or, at the very least, reduce the resting level of activity to below the pain threshold activation level. In order to evaluate whether this might be possible within the scope of clinical dental practice for any individual patient requires an in depth assessment of the pain history from its first appearance to the present day, so that the factors generating ongoing neural activity can be weighted to determine whether those amenable to dental intervention might produce sufficient effect. In the case of a patient whose child had died no amount of dental intervention would resolve the chronic pain perceived for years in the upper canine region since this patient was edentulous and therefore the diagnosis of psychosocially generated activity maintaining the central sensitization was made; that is "psychosocial allodynia". In this case the appropriate course of action was to guide the patient toward a psychological/psychiatric solution. In another patient complete resolution of their headaches was effected when the chewing of gum was ceased, highlighting the contribution of physical factors in this case.

The majority of patients fit between these two extremes. Clinical observation suggests that the greater the physical factors which contribute to the ongoing neural activity, the more amenable is the pain to be relieved through physical intervention. Conversely, the greater the psychosocial contribution, the less likely that physical intervention will ameliorate the pain, and for some people such intervention may even exacerbate the situation.

Another factor that requires careful consideration is the patient's "readiness to move on". Highlighting this are the histories of two patients. The first, a patient who presented for routine dental treatment and did not reveal their history of multiple episodes of severe chronic pain that followed routine dental treatment, even when asked explicitly during the pretreatment evaluation. The history was reluctantly and selectively revealed over subsequent visits as the pre-existing pain exacerbated. After sufficient information was gleaned to proffer an approach that might provide effective management the patient's response was "don't go there"; an example of 'not ready to move on'. The second patient presented with severe, unremitting head and neck pain that had persisted over a number of years. The history provided included two separate abusive spousal relationships and a third in which the spouse was gentle and loving; this latter spouse was suffering from terminal cancer. After addressing the psychosocial component through discussion and instruction in a simple breathing/relaxation/meditation technique, about two weeks later at the subsequent appointment, the patient reported that the pain had diminished by ninety per cent. At this visit occlusal adjustment was undertaken in an attempt to address a physical factor contributing to resting neural activity and at the subsequent visit the pain was completely resolved; this patient was "ready to move on".

These two examples highlight the clinician's ethical responsibility to respect each individual patient's autonomy. It can be argued that by respecting the former patient's choice of "don't go there" and "not ready to move on" the clinician's duty of care was fulfilled even though the patient remained in pain.

There is controversy surrounding occlusal adjustment as a valid treatment in relieving persistent (chronic) head and neck pain. A morphologically (anatomical or anatomo-physiological) based rationale for the effectiveness of occlusal adjustment does not stand up to rigorous scientific investigation. Any "one size fits all" morphological formula cannot, therefore, provide the explanation for, or guidance to effective pain management with this tool. However, the clinician-scientist's neuroscientific explanation for the effectiveness of occlusal adjustment in bringing pain relief may be drawn from the research of Trulsson and Johansson on the force/activity relationship of human periodontal mechanoreceptor afferents, including the effect of force direction, reported in the literature in articles dating from 1992 [9 - 15]. In 80-85% of the receptors a hyperbolic relationship was exhibited with progressive loading of the teeth, the greatest change in activity being induced with the early lightest force and with negligible activity increase beyond a certain force level irrespective of increased loading. The clinical observation that when adjusting an occlusion the difference between pain and its resolution is a fraction of a millimeter may be explained by this loading characteristic. It also explains the discomfort associated with a "high" filling; the associated pain might be described as examples of "occlusal allodynia". [An analogous neural mechanism may underlie the relief obtained when removing a small stone from the sole of one's shoe]. This research provides a neuroscientific model of occlusion free from the morphological variations that plague the debate on what constitutes an optimal/ideal occlusion and sets the aim of occlusal adjustment in terms of neural activity reduction. The resulting occlusal morphological schema associated with an optimal occlusion will be unique to each individual: an optimal occlusion might then be defined as the occlusal schema for any individual that induces the lowest level of neural activity for that individual with the teeth in centric occlusion (maximum interdigitation). Such conceptualization is consistent with a personalized rather than population approach to patient management. Until now only neural activity, whether the source is psychosocial or physical has been discussed in relation to pain. The findings of psycho-neuroimmunology research (the study of neuro-immun--endocrine interactions) enable and demand an expanded consideration. Study of neuro-immune-endocrine interactions has shown the seamless intra-, extra-, and inter-cellular communication between these traditionally thought of separate systems, reintegrating them into the unified neuro-immuno-endocrine network, where activity in one is activity in all [1, 16 - 31]. Therefore, it would follow that the principles of one are the principles of all a unified systems biomedical understanding where activity in any one of the traditionally defined systems may be expressed in any other, singly or in combination. The message that the messenger pain is relaying, therefore, may relate to any area of this network, at least theoretically. A clinical observation supporting this was the case of a female patient in my practice suffering from unremitting, unresponsive orofacial pain for a number of years, who experienced considerable relief when the brand of contraceptive pill (and estrogen component) she was taking was changed.

CONCLUSION

A working clinical model of pain (including orofacial pain) might then define pain as being a centrally mediated perception; a messenger warning that something is amiss. This message might be deciphered by following rigorous diagnostic protocols and procedures. Whether acute or persistent (chronic) the message pertains to ongoing activity, generated by physical and/or psychosocial sources, at a level above the pain threshold. Beyond the conceptual artificial boundaries of the traditional divisions of biomedicine, the activity can arise from anywhere in the neuro-immuno-endocrine network and it is the net sum of all the activity of this network by which pain is generated. Rather than assuming idiopathic pain to be pathological, defining it as "unexplained" leaves open the possibility of future explanation, whilst allowing the clinical focus to be on the strategies for its relief. This might be achieved even without the knowledge of the pathology or imbalance that the pain (messenger) is warning of, if the net level of total activity can be reduced to below the pain threshold irrespective of the origin of the activity reduction.

PART 2

The Clinician Detective: Applying the Clinician's Journey to Patient Management.

My personal approach to implement the understandings derived from the clinician's journey to patient management requires me to undertake a comprehensive analysis and diagnosis of each patient's individual condition and circumstance. This is achieved through seven systematic steps summarised under the following headings:

1. Presenting concern
2. History and course of the concern
3. Medical history
4. Personal history
5. Examination
6. Diagnosis / Differential diagnosis
7. Treatment options

Effective pain management requires a personalised patient centred approach where listening is at least as important as any other investigation. Central to this is recording a comprehensive, non-judgemental history. My initial question relates to the presenting complaint; *e.g.* "What is your concern?", "How can I help you?", "What brought you here today?" Interpreting what a patient is saying requires listening with ears, eyes, and professional experience and intuition. Often cues are provided in non-verbal ways *via* body-language, gestures, hesitations and tones. If it is established that pain is primary to or associated with the patient's concern then its history and course are sought *e.g.* "When did it first appear?", "What was happening (in your life) at the time?", "How long did the pain last?", "Has it been intermittent or continuous since then?", "How frequent are the episodes and how long do they last?", "Does anything make the pain better?", "Does anything make the pain worse?", "What sort of pain do you feel?", "How severe is the pain?".

By listening to the patient's story I assure the patient that mine is a personalised, patient centred approach and his/her being in pain is believed and taken seriously.

This often provides the patient with the confidence to share more deeply and more personally.

A comprehensive medical history provides essential information that enables both the inclusion and exclusion of current and historical factors that might be contributing to the patient's pain. Although much of the information is gained through a formal questionnaire (written and verbal), many patients provide additional and significant medical (and other) information throughout the appointment (and even at subsequent appointments). Sometimes this is because they think that the information is irrelevant, whilst at other times patients conceal the information which is of a more personal nature until their confidence is sufficient for them to reveal further.

History taking might be thought analogous to piecing a jig-saw puzzle, where the relevant pieces appear in a semi-random manner.

It is important to ascertain each patient's personal circumstances, both current and historical, to elucidate any relevant stressors; *e.g.* "What do you do during the day?", "Do you have children?", "Do you have a partner?", "Do you have a family?", "Do you have friends around you?", "Do you enjoy your job?", "Do you sleep well and how many hours do you sleep each night?", "Do you have support for the things you do?", "What stresses you?", "When do you get time out?", "How do you relax?", "Do you get time for yourself?" … one question leads to another often providing insight into a host of physical and/or psychosocial factors that might be contributing to the patient's condition. Physical examination and relevant testing are then undertaken.

The total information accumulated provides the basis for the provisional or definitive diagnosis including an assessment of the ratio of physical to psychosocial factors contributing towards the pain. When a definitive diagnosis cannot be established as to the source(s) of the patient's pain then, in the orofacial pain clinic, the patient might be offered a series of treatment steps (commencing with the least invasive or that thought most likely to address the pain) aimed at eliminating potential sources.

Treatment options offered will depend on the ratio of physical to psychosocial source contribution and are tailored to each patient's circumstances as described in Part 1. Sometimes the source of pain cannot be directly addressed and an indirect strategy that reduces the overall neural/biomedical activity may be suggested in the hope that this might lower the overall system activity to below the pain threshold switch-on level. At other times it is beyond my scope of practice and the patient is referred to a more appropriate care provider. Throughout each appointment, I attempt to respect the patient's autonomy and their choices in a non-judgemental manner, accepting their right to provide whatever information they care to share and treatment they care to accept or refuse.

CONFILICT OF INTERST

The authors confirm that they have no conflict of interest to declare for this publication.

ACKNOWLEDGEMENT

Declared none.

REFERENCES

[1] Besedovsky HO, Rey AD. Physiology of psychoneuroimmunology: a personal view. Brain Behav Immun 2007; 21(1): 34-44.
[http://dx.doi.org/10.1016/j.bbi.2006.09.008] [PMID: 17157762]

[2] Moffat B. A biological consideration of centric relation based on skeletal and connective tissue responses. In: Celenza FV, Nasedkin JN, Eds. Occlusion: the state of the art. Chicago, Illinois 1978; pp. 13-8.

[3] Woolf CJ. Central sensitization: implications for the diagnosis and treatment of pain. Pain 2011; 152(3) (Suppl.): S2-S15.
[http://dx.doi.org/10.1016/j.pain.2010.09.030] [PMID: 20961685]

[4] Basser DS. Chronic pain: a neuroscientific understanding. Med Hypotheses 2012; 78(1): 79-85.
[http://dx.doi.org/10.1016/j.mehy.2011.09.045] [PMID: 22019262]

[5] Basbaum AI, Jessell TM. The Perception of Pain. In: Kandel ER, Schwartz JH, Jessell TM, Eds. The principles of neural science. 4th ed. McGraw-Hill 2000; pp. 472-91.

[6] Latremoliere A, Woolf CJ. Central sensitization: a generator of pain hypersensitivity by central neural plasticity. J Pain 2009; 10(9): 895-926.
[http://dx.doi.org/10.1016/j.jpain.2009.06.012] [PMID: 19712899]

[7] Ren K, Dubner R. Central nervous system plasticity and persistent pain. J Orofac Pain 1999; 13(3): 155-63.
[PMID: 10823030]

[8] Schur EA, Afari N, Furberg H, *et al.* Feeling bad in more ways than one: comorbidity patterns of medically unexplained and psychiatric conditions. J Gen Intern Med 2007; 22(6): 818-21. [http://dx.doi.org/10.1007/s11606-007-0140-5] [PMID: 17503107]

[9] Trulsson M, Johansson RS, Olsson KA. Directional sensitivity of human periodontal mechanoreceptive afferents to forces applied to the teeth. J Physiol 1992; 447: 373-89. [http://dx.doi.org/10.1113/jphysiol.1992.sp019007] [PMID: 1593451]

[10] Trulsson M. Multiple-tooth receptive fields of single human periodontal mechanoreceptive afferents. J Neurophysiol 1993; 69(2): 474-81. [PMID: 8459279]

[11] Trulsson M, Johansson RS. Encoding of amplitude and rate of forces applied to the teeth by human periodontal mechanoreceptive afferents. J Neurophysiol 1994; 72(4): 1734-44. [PMID: 7823098]

[12] Trulsson M, Johansson RS. Encoding of tooth loads by human periodontal afferents and their role in jaw motor control. Prog Neurobiol 1996; 49(3): 267-84. [http://dx.doi.org/10.1016/S0301-0082(96)00016-0] [PMID: 8878305]

[13] Trulsson M. Sensory and motor function of teeth and dental implants: a basis for osseoperception. Clin Exp Pharmacol Physiol 2005; 32(1-2): 119-22. [http://dx.doi.org/10.1111/j.1440-1681.2005.04139.x] [PMID: 15730446]

[14] Johnsen SE, Trulsson M. Encoding of amplitude and rate of tooth loads by human periodontal afferents from premolar and molar teeth. J Neurophysiol 2005; 93(4): 1889-97. [http://dx.doi.org/10.1152/jn.00664.2004] [PMID: 15563554]

[15] Trulsson M. Sensory-motor function of human periodontal mechanoreceptors. J Oral Rehabil 2006; 33(4): 262-73. [http://dx.doi.org/10.1111/j.1365-2842.2006.01629.x] [PMID: 16629881]

[16] Ader R, Kelley KW. A global view of twenty years of Brain, Behavior, and Immunity. Brain Behav Immun 2007; 21(1): 20-2. [http://dx.doi.org/10.1016/j.bbi.2006.07.003] [PMID: 16996715]

[17] Blalock JE, Smith EM. Conceptual development of the immune system as a sixth sense. Brain Behav Immun 2007; 21(1): 23-33. [http://dx.doi.org/10.1016/j.bbi.2006.09.004] [PMID: 17088044]

[18] Dantzer R, Kelley KW. Twenty years of research on cytokine-induced sickness behavior. Brain Behav Immun 2007; 21(2): 153-60. [http://dx.doi.org/10.1016/j.bbi.2006.09.006] [PMID: 17088043]

[19] Malarkey WB, Mills PJ. Endocrinology: the active partner in PNI research. Brain Behav Immun 2007; 21(2): 161-8. [http://dx.doi.org/10.1016/j.bbi.2006.10.008] [PMID: 17174524]

[20] Bonneau RH, Padgett DA, Sheridan JF. Twenty years of psychoneuroimmunology and viral infections in Brain, Behavior, and Immunity. Brain Behav Immun 2007; 21(3): 273-80. [http://dx.doi.org/10.1016/j.bbi.2006.10.004] [PMID: 17158025]

[21] Gosselin D, Rivest S. Role of IL-1 and TNF in the brain: twenty years of progress on a Dr. Jekyll/Mr. Hyde duality of the innate immune system. Brain Behav Immun 2007; 21(3): 281-9. [http://dx.doi.org/10.1016/j.bbi.2006.12.004] [PMID: 17275255]

[22] Irwin MR, Miller AH. Depressive disorders and immunity: 20 years of progress and discovery. Brain Behav Immun 2007; 21(4): 374-83. [http://dx.doi.org/10.1016/j.bbi.2007.01.010] [PMID: 17360153]

[23] Kelley KW, Weigent DA, Kooijman R. Protein hormones and immunity. Brain Behav Immun 2007; 21(4): 384-92. [http://dx.doi.org/10.1016/j.bbi.2006.11.010] [PMID: 17198749]

[24] Straub RH. Autoimmune disease and innervation. Brain Behav Immun 2007; 21(5): 528-34. [http://dx.doi.org/10.1016/j.bbi.2007.04.005] [PMID: 17517488]

[25] Goehler LE, Lyte M, Gaykema RP. Infection-induced viscerosensory signals from the gut enhance anxiety: implications for psychoneuroimmunology. Brain Behav Immun 2007; 21(6): 721-6. [http://dx.doi.org/10.1016/j.bbi.2007.02.005] [PMID: 17428636]

[26] Quan N, Banks WA. Brain-immune communication pathways. Brain Behav Immun 2007; 21(6): 727-35. [http://dx.doi.org/10.1016/j.bbi.2007.05.005] [PMID: 17604598]

[27] Nance DM, Sanders VM. Autonomic innervation and regulation of the immune system (1987-2007). Brain Behav Immun 2007; 21(6): 736-45. [http://dx.doi.org/10.1016/j.bbi.2007.03.008] [PMID: 17467231]

[28] Moynihan JA, Santiago FM. Brain behavior and immunity: twenty years of T cells. Brain Behav Immun 2007; 21(7): 872-80. [http://dx.doi.org/10.1016/j.bbi.2007.06.010] [PMID: 17681745]

[29] Ben-Eliyahu S, Page GG, Schleifer SJ. Stress, NK cells, and cancer: Still a promissory note. Brain Behav Immun 2007; 21(7): 881-7. [http://dx.doi.org/10.1016/j.bbi.2007.06.008] [PMID: 17662574]

[30] Coe CL, Laudenslager ML. Psychosocial influences on immunity, including effects on immune maturation and senescence. Brain Behav Immun 2007; 21(8): 1000-8. [http://dx.doi.org/10.1016/j.bbi.2007.06.015] [PMID: 17706917]

[31] Kemeny ME, Schedlowski M. Understanding the interaction between psychosocial stress and immune-related diseases: a stepwise progression. Brain Behav Immun 2007; 21(8): 1009-18. [http://dx.doi.org/10.1016/j.bbi.2007.07.010] [PMID: 17889502]

CHAPTER 2

Functional Brain Circuitry in Central Post-stroke Pain

Andrew Chih Wei Huang[1], **Hsiang-Chin Lu**[2] and **Bai Chuang Shyu**[2,*]

[1] *Department of Psychology, Fo Guang University, Yilan, Taiwan, Republic of China*

[2] *Institute of Biomedical Sciences, Academia Sinica, Taipei, Taiwan, Republic of China*

Abstract: Central post-stroke pain (CPSP) results from lesions or dysfunction of the spinothalamocortical pathway. Pathophysiological mechanism of CPSP may include contralateral somatosensory cortex or bilateral mid- and posterior insula, anterior insula, posterior cingulate cortex and spinothalamocortical pathway. Our [^{14}C] iodoantipyrine data from animal model of CPSP indicated that significantly higher activation occurs in the medial prefrontal cortex (mPFC), anterior cingulate cortex, thalamus, hypothalamus, amygdala and periaqueductal gray (PAG). We propose a neural correlation hypothesis of CPSP, in which the mPFC-amygdala pathway, hypothalamus and PAG interact with each other and the spinothalamocortical pathway, resulting in the manifestation of CPSP symptoms. These symptoms can include depression, anxiety, motor disturbances and cognitive dysfunction in thalamic stroke patients, in addition to CPSP. Alterations in different brain activation and circuitry connections in CPSP may help in understanding the pathophysiological mechanisms underlying multiple aspects of CPSP symptoms. Such novel ideas may be applied to develop pharmacological and non-pharmacological interventions for CPSP.

Keywords: CPSP, Nociceptive stimuli, Spinothalamocprtical pathway.

INTRODUCTION

Based on the definition of the International Association for the Study of Pain, central pain is attributable to primary lesions or dysfunction of the central nervous system [1]. The clinical characteristics of central pain are severely confounded by

* **Coresponding author Bai Chuang Shyu:** Institute of Biomedical Sciences, Academia Sinica, Taipei, Taiwan, Republic of China; Email: bmbai@gate.sinica.edu.tw

Puneetpal Singh (Ed.)

the characteristics of peripheral pain, with the exception of the location of neuropathic damage in the central or peripheral nervous system [2]. Distinguishing between central pain and peripheral pain is important, in which damage or dysfunction of spinothalamocortical mechanisms is critical for central pain but not peripheral pain [3]. Despite the distinctions between central and peripheral pain, "deafferentation pain" is suggested to be common to both central and peripheral pain. Both types of pain involve deficits or decreases in sensory inputs to the nervous system; thus, they share some clinical characteristics [4]. The essential characteristics of central pain consist of dysesthesia or paresthesia, persistent or paroxysmal pain, and spontaneous or evoked pain. When central pain is caused by stroke, with damage or dysfunction of the central nervous system, central pain is referred to as central post-stroke pain (CPSP) [5].

1. CLINICAL SYMPTOMS OF CENTRAL POST-STROKE PAIN

Previous studies thought that CPSP results from thalamic lesions, referred to as thalamic symptoms [6]. However, recent findings have shown that CPSP is also associated with extra-thalamic lesions [7]. The prevalence of CPSP is uncertain. Klit *et al.* [6] reported prevalence between 1% and 12% whereas another study reported it to be 8-35% [5]. Although the prevalence of CPSP is diverse, it appears to be > 8% in stroke patients. The cardinal symptoms of CPSP include pain that is attributable to impairments in the spinothalamocortical pathway. This impairment of the spinothalamocortical circuitry is resulted in the neuropathic pain. In general, peripheral sensitization and central sensitization are two major neuronal mechanisms underlying the neuropathic pain. Previous evidences have reported that the noxious stimuli may sensitize the peripheral nervous structure resulted in sensitization development, wind-up or expansion of receptive fields of nociceptive neurons. Moreover, molecules such as prostaglandin and bradykinin have been seen as pain mediators to affect peripheral sensitization and peripheral pain. These molecules are resulted from the tissue damage or inflammation, and they are suggested to involve peripheral sensitization and hyper-activation from peripheral signaling of sensory neurons. CPSP is primarily due to the central sensitization mechanism. Hyper-excitability of the central neuronal circuitry in the central pain involves abnormal neurotransmission of glutamate, substance P and nitric oxide. Central sensitization can be reduced by the brain GABA receptor agonism or the glutamate (such as NMDA) receptor antagonism. GABA or NMDA categories of drugs have been developed to treat CPSP patients. For example, carbamazepine, which was a typical antiepileptic drug and GABA receptor agonist, are frequently used to reduce abnormal hyperactivity for the involvement of central neuronal disinhibition. Ketamine is another treatment method for CPSP that is one of NMDA receptor antagonists. It was evident that intravenous ketamine administration can effectively reduce the CPSP symptom. In addition, oral administrations of ketamine can alleviate dysphoria when using to combine with oral diazepam. On the other hand, pain perception may be spontaneous or evoked. In spontaneous pain, some cases present a continuous way and some are shown a paroxysmal way. Regardless of continuous or paroxysmal conditions, patients with CPSP often suffer from sensations of burning, aching, squeezing, pricking, lacerating, shooting, throbbing, heaviness, and cold. Evoked pain in CPSP is caused by nociceptive or non-nociceptive stimuli. Nociceptive stimuli can induce hyperalgesia in punctuate and thermal conditions. Non-nociceptive stimuli elicit allodynia in thermal, static, and dynamic conditions. Therefore, allodynia and hyperalgesia are likely important features of CPSP symptoms.

In addition to pain symptoms, some psychological, social, and physiological functions are also impaired in patients who suffer from stroke hemorrhage and consequently CPSP [8]. For example, previous studies showed that stroke hemorrhage patients may present motor dysfunction and clinical depression [9, 10]. Patients with stroke hemorrhage have been shown to present affective and apathetic symptoms, such as anxiety and depression [11]. Moreover, clinical data have shown that patients with thalamic lesions exhibited cognitive dysfunction [12]. After focal thalamic lesions, explicit memory and implicit memory can also be impaired [13]. Moreover, amnesia was present following thalamic hemorrhage [14]. Quality of life and motivation also deteriorate after stroke. Patients with CPSP may present blunting of thought processes that affects mood and intellect and produces neurotic tendencies [15]. Additionally, patients with CPSP have an increased risk of suicide associated with loss of sleep, libido, and appetite [16]. Poor social interactions and an inability to work have also been found in such patients. In conclusion, pain symptoms are an essential component of CPSP, but such patients often also exhibit multiple impairments or symptoms in the psychological, social, and physiological domains.

2. PATHOGENESIS-RELATED HYPOTHESES OF CENTRAL POST-STROKE PAIN

The pathogenesis of CPSP has been reported to involve dysfunction of the spinothalamocortical pathway [17]. Impairments in any of the neural substrates of the spinothalamocortical pathway can induce CPSP symptoms. The symptoms of CPSP may result from lesions of the spinal cord [18], thalamus [19], and cortical areas [20, 21]. Some hypotheses have been proposed, including central disinhibition, central imbalance of stimuli, and central sensitization, to explain many aspects of the pathogenesis of CPSP.

2.1. Central Disinhibition

In 1911, Head and Holmes suggested that stroke patients with damage in the lateral thalamus presented disinhibition in the medial thalamus, resulting in pain. In their study, they found that injury of the spinothalamocortical pathway caused CPSP symptoms to emerge [22]. This viewpoint is supported by central inhibition from the lateral thalamus to medial thalamus, which can cause sensations of burning, cold, and ongoing pain and allodynia [19]. Therefore, the sensory deficit for CPSP patients is found for the perception of cold and heat, cotton whip, and vibration. Moreover, discriminative sensory deficits can occur, and CPSP patients may experience allodynia or hyperalgesia in response to evoked pain that is caused by central disinhibition [19].

2.2. Central Imbalance

Central imbalance was proposed based on the dissociated sensory loss that is observed in CPSP. CPSP patients often report that they have normal touch and vibration sensations, but their pain and temperature perceptions are abnormal [5]. Therefore, central imbalance appears to occur from the dissociated loss of different sensory modalities. For example, laser-evoked heat stimulation at different sites on the body was employed to examine the influence of different sensations on cerebral electrical potentials. The results showed that cerebral potentials changed in response to the laser stimulus that caused pain and temperature sensations, but cerebral potentials were unaffected by mechano stimulation [23]. The occurrence of pain and dysesthesia are attributable to central imbalance between the dorsal column of the spinal cord and spinothalamocortical pathway. This means that deficits in the spinothalamocortical system produce loss inputs to the spared dorsal and medial lemniscus of spinal cord, and thereby there is no interaction from the spinothalamocortical system to the spared dorsal and medial lemniscus. Therefore, it produces central imbalance that causes dysesthesia and central pain [24].

2.3. Central Sensitization

The central sensitization hypothesis proposes that lesions of neurons in the central nervous system result in the loss of inhibitory neuron inputs and enhance the excitability of surrounding neurons, thereby producing central pain, termed central sensitization [6]. Some electrophysiological studies have provided empirical evidence to support the central sensitization hypothesis, in which central nociceptive neurons can control allodynia, spontaneous pain, or evoked pain [25 - 28]. An electrophysiological and positron emission tomography (PET) study found that the analgesic effect of precentral gyrus stimulation (*i.e.*, a treatment for refractory post-stroke pain) was associated with the facilitation of synaptic activity in the thalamus and brainstem [27]. Spontaneous pain was highly correlated with spontaneous hyperactivity in the dorsal region of the spinal cord and ventral posterior thalamus that was attributable to deafferentation [28]. An electrophysiological clinical human study found that following central neuropathic pain, the threshold of calcium spike bursts in the thalamus decreased, thereby eliciting neurogenic pain or other positive symptoms [25]. Moreover, spontaneous neuronal activity in the thalamic principle sensory nucleus was shown to result in pain perception or dysesthesia in patients with spinal cord transection [26]. Therefore, the central sensitization hypothesis focuses on neuronal hyperexcitability that underlies deafferentation following lesions or dysfunction of the central nervous system.

In summary, the current central disinhibition, central imbalance, and central sensitization hypotheses do not conflict with each other. Each of them emphasizes a specific component of central pain and dysesthesia. Central disinhibition stresses that central pain is attributable to disinhibition of the connection between the lateral thalamus and medial thalamus following lesions or dysfunction of the spinothalamocortical pathway. Central imbalance emphasizes that lesions and dysfunction of the spinothalamocortical system diminish sensory inputs to the spared dorsal and medial lemniscus of spinal cord, and thereby induce imbalance of the interaction from the spinothalamocortical system to the spared dorsal and medial lemniscus of spinal cord. Thus, it causes dysesthesia and central pain. Central sensitization emphasizes that neural hyperactivity occurs following lesions or damage of any neural substrate of the spinothalamocortical pathway and causes central pain. Fig. (**1**) shows the relationships between these three hypotheses to explain the occurrence of CPSP.

3. FUNCTIONAL BRAIN ACTIVITY MAPPING

3.1. Human Neuroimaging of Central Post-stroke Pain

A growing body of brain mapping evidence has shown that various neural substrates are involved in central pain in patients following stroke and in patients who do not experience stroke [29]. The data have been diverse, and few studies have failed to support the concept of the pain matrix [30]. The pain matrix has been found to be widespread and distributed in many brain areas, including the contralateral somatosensory cortex and bilateral mid- and posterior insula, anterior insula, and posterior cingulate cortex mediate pain perception [31]. The pain matrix in the cortex is conceptually a crucial neural substrate for pain processing in the brain.

Many previous studies have demonstrated the involvement of specific brain areas in CPSP, with lesions or dysfunction of the spinothalamocortical pathway. For example, using a human model, Craig *et al.* [32] performed PET to manipulate noxious cold and heat stimuli and compared cortical activation patterns associated with thermal pain, indicating that the anterior cingulate cortex plays an important role in CPSP. In a functional magnetic resonance imaging (fMRI) study, Ducreux *et al.* [30] employed a pathological model, Syringomyelia, and cold or brush-evoked allodynia and found that different types of allodynia have different neural substrates. However, the authors reported that these different brain areas that are involved in pain processing were not fully consistent with the pain matrix [30]. A PET study [33] used [^{15}O]-labeled water during electrical nociceptive stimulation and [^{18}F] fluorodeoxyglucose to assess brain metabolism. They found that particular neural substrates were activated, including the posterior insula, secondary somatosensory cortex, postcentral gyrus, and primary somatosensory cortex. A human fMRI study [34] utilized noxious heat and cold stimuli to evoke pain and found that the anterior cingulate cortex, ventral portion of the posterior cingulate cortex, and supplementary motor area were activated in central pain. Another PET study administered [^{11}C] diprenorphine, an opioid receptor antagonist, in patients with CPSP or peripheral pain. They found a significant reduction of opioid receptor binding in the posterior midbrain, medial thalamus and insula, and temporal and prefrontal cortices [35]. A similar [^{11}C] diprenorphine PET study found a significant decrease in opioid receptor binding in the contralateral thalamus, parietal cortex, secondary somatosensory cortex, insula, lateral prefrontal cortex (PFC), anterior and posterior cingulate cortex, and midbrain gray matter [36]. A brain mapping study of chronic migraine pain provided evidence that the dorsal rostral pons, anterior cingulate cortex, and cuneus were correlated with pain perception when electrical stimulation was applied to primary sensory inputs [37]. Moreover, a recent fMRI study employed diffusion tensor imaging to assess activation patterns in the pain network and thalamocortical tract. The results showed that a pain reduction therapy, repetitive transcranial magnetic stimulation, decreased activation in the secondary somatosensory cortex, insula, prefrontal cortex, and putamen [38]. A human fMRI study [39] used nociceptive stimulation to induce pain. The results showed that some cerebral structures were activated, including the thalamus, somatosensory cortex, insula, and anterior cingulate cortex. Another fMRI study was performed with different thermal nociceptive stimuli to evoke pain and examined the neural substrates that are involved in CPSP symptoms. Their data showed that the anterior cingulate gyrus and parietal association cortex were active [21]. Another study [40] performed an fMRI study and reported that the contralateral thalamus, S1 cortex, bilateral S2 cortex, anterior and posterior insula, mid-anterior cingulate cortex, and supplemental motor area might control C-fiber-evoked pain responses. Symonds *et al.* also performed an fMRI study with acute pain stimuli to elucidate the involvement of specific brain areas. The cortical "pain matrix" (*i.e.*, contralateral somatosensory cortex, bilateral mid/posterior insula, anterior insula, and posterior cingulate gyrus) was strongly active in response to acute pain [31] (Table **1**).

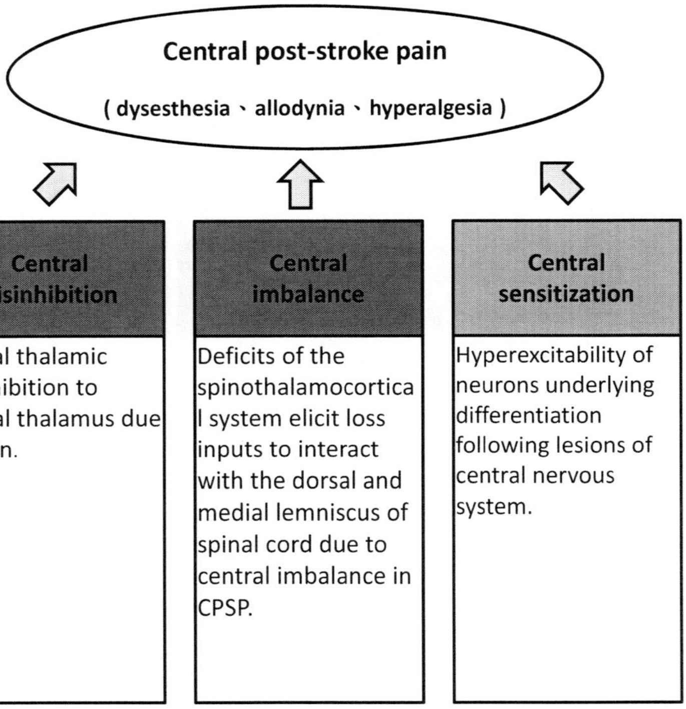

Fig. (1). Three hypotheses of CPSP: central disinhibition, central imbalance, and central sensitization.

In summary, human brain imaging data show that the neural substrates of CPSP are diverse. Nevertheless, the cortical pain matrix (*e.g.*, contralateral somatosensory cortex, bilateral mid and posterior insula, anterior insula, and posterior cingulate cortex) appears to mediate pain processing in CPSP patients.

Table 1. Brain mapping in central neuropathic pain following stroke.

Authors & years	Method	Subjects	Conduction	Findings
Craig *et al.* (1996)	PET	Human	Conduct noxious cold & heat stimuli to compare the cortical activation patterns for thermal pain.	Anterior cingulate cortex.
Dureux *et al.* (2006)	fMRI	Human	Syringomyelia: a pathological model.	Different types of allodynia exhibit to different brain activities, but it does not respond to "pain matrix".
			With cold or blush-evoked allodynia.	Distinct pathophysiological mechanisms are associated to the different modalities of allodynia.
Kassubek *et al.* (2003)	PET	Human	Using ^{15}O-labelled water during electrical nociceptive stimulation.	Posterior insula.
			^{18}F-fluorodeoxyglucose (FDG) □ a brain metabolism.	Secondary somatosensory cortex.
				Postcentral gyrus / primary somatosensory cortex.
Kwan *et al.* (2000)	fMRI	Human	Noxious heat & cold stimuli.	Anterior cingulate cortex.
			Innocuous cool & warm stimuli.	Ventral portion of the posterior cingulate cortex.
				Supplementary motor area.
Maarawi *et al.* (2007)	PET	Human	Using PET & [^{11}C]diprenorphine for cpsp & peripheral pain.	A significant decrease in opioid binding in posterior midbrain, medial thalamus and insular, temporal & prefrontal cortices to pain.
Matharu *et al.* (2003)	PET	Human	Using electrical stimulation of primary sensory input to assess an antinociceptive effect.	Dorsal rostral pons correlated
				ACC & cuneus to pain
Ohn *et al.* (2013)	fMRI & DTI	Human	Using diffusion tensor imaging (DTI) and fMRI to asses the activation patterns of the pain network and the thalamocortical tract.	Secondary somatosensory cortex.
				Insula, prefrontal cortex, and putamen.

(Table 1) contd.....

Authors & years	Method	Subjects	Conduction	Findings
Rainville *et al.* (2001)	fMRI	Human	Nociceptive stimulation evoked pain.	.Cerebral structure including thalamus, the somatosensory, insular, and anterior cingulate cortices.
Seghier *et al.* (2005)	fMRI & DTI	Human	Using different thermonociceptive stimuli to assess the brain areas for pain.	Anterior cingulate gyrus & the associative parietal regions.
Staud *et al* (2007)	fMRI	Human	Using temporal summation of second pain to assess the brain areas due to c-fiber-evoked responses.	Contralateral thalamus.
				S1.
				Bilateral S2, anterior and posterior insula.
				Mid-anterior cingulate cortex.
				Supplement motor area.
Symonds *et al.* (2006)	fMRI	Human	Using acute pain stimuli to assess the involvements of brain areas.	Cortical "pain matrix" includes contralateral somatosensory cortex, bilaterally mid/posterior insula, anterior insula, and posterior cingulate cortex.
Willoch *et al.* (2004)	PET	Human	Using PET & [^{11}C]diprenorphine.	Reduced [11C] diprenorphine opioid binding in contralateral thalamus, parietal, secondary somatosensory, insular and lateral prefrontal cortices.
				Anterior and posterior cingulate cortex.
				Midbrain gray matter.
Hess *et al.* (2007)	fMRI	Animal	Temperature stimulations at the hindpaw to assess the brain areas in pain.	Cingulate, retrosplenial, sensory-motor and insular cortex, medial and lateral posterior thalamus.
				Pretectal area, hypothalamus, periagueductal grey.
Jiang *et al.* (2014)	fMRI	Animal	Using motor cortex stimulations can reduce pain.	Primary somatosensory cortex.
				Prefrontal cortex.

3.2. Animal Neuroimaging of CPSP

In contrast to human models, little animal research has evaluated the neural substrates of CPSP symptoms, but the available animal brain mapping data are seemingly consistent with human data [41, 42]. For example, thermal stimulation of the hindpaws was employed to assess the involvement of specific brain areas and activation in the cingulate cortex, retrosplenial cortex, sensory-motor cortex, insula, and medial and lateral posterior thalamus was observed. Moreover, pain processing appeared to involve the pretectal area, hypothalamus, and periaqueductal gray (PAG) [41]. Additionally, motor cortex stimulation was applied to reduce pain and showed that changes in brain activation occurred in the primary somatosensory cortex and PFC [42]. Altogether, the animal brain mapping data for CPSP were similar to those reported in human models of CPSP.

3.3. [^{14}C] Iodoantipyrine Data and Region-of-Interest Analysis of CPSP in Animal Models

Recently, we used [^{14}C] iodoantipyrine (IAP) to assess the neural substrates that are involved in CPSP in an animal model with lesions of the ventrobasal complex in the right thalamus and evaluate the ways in which these neural substrates are connected with each other. Based on [^{14}C] IAP brain mapping, brain activity was positively correlated with the [^{14}C] IAP signal intensity. The brain image pixel intensity of [^{14}C] IAP labeling reflects metabolism in the brain, which can then be quantitatively analyzed. Following lesions of the ventrobasal complex, we found that rats in the CPSP group exhibited a shorter withdrawal time from thermal pain in the plantar test, with a decrease in the threshold of mechanical force in the von Frey test (Fig. **2A, B**).

The results indicated that lesions of the ventrobasal complex in the right thalamus evoked CPSP symptoms, including behavioral hyperalgesia, in thermal and mechanical pain. Furthermore, the signal intensities of the brain images were normalized and analyzed by statistical parametric mapping (SPM). The data of the pixel count ratio of SMP showed that activation of the cortex, striatum, thalamus, hypothalamus, and amygdala was significantly enhanced in the CPSP group compared with the sham group. However, the ventrobasal complex in the thalamus presented lower activation in the CPSP group (Fig. **3**).

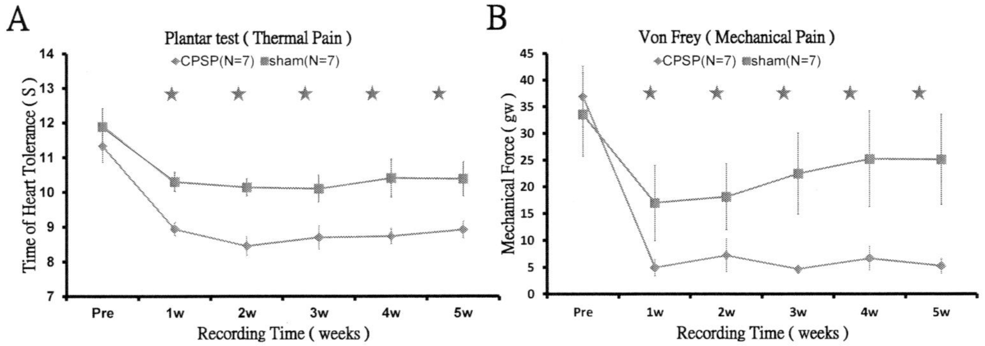

Fig. (2). Example of mechanical and thermal hyperalgesia after lesions of the ventrobasal complex in the thalamus. **(A)**. The plantar test and (B). von Frey test were performed on the left hindpaw in the sham and CPSP groups on day 35. (*) indicates, $p < 0.05$. The results showed that the CPSP group had lower pain thresholds than the sham group. Adapted from Lu *et al.* [39].

Additionally, a region-of-interest (ROI) analysis was conducted based on the radioactivity ratio, which was transformed from the raw pixel intensity data. Possible brain areas to involve pain mechanisms were determined and labeled (Fig. **4A**). The results revealed significant differences in the infralimbic cortex, cingulate cortex area 1 (Cg1), motor cortex area 2 (M2), dorsal agranular insular cortex (AID), ventral agranular insular cortex (AIV), hippocampus-3, and PAG in the left hemisphere between the CPSP and sham groups (Fig. **4B**). The right hemisphere presented significant differences in the radioactivity ratio in the infralimbic cortex, prelimbic cortex, Cg1-1, ventrobasal complex, and amygdala-2 (Fig. **4C**).

Overall, the SPM and ROI analysis results indicated that activation of the infralimbic cortex, prelimbic cortex, Cg1, M2, S1, granular insular cortex, AID, AIV, hippocampus, mediodorsal thalamic nucleus, ventrobasal complex, ventrolateral thalamus nucleus, ventromedial thalamic nucleus, lateral hypothalamus, ventromedial hypothalamic nucleus, amygdala, and PAG was significantly different between the CPSP and sham groups (Table **2**).

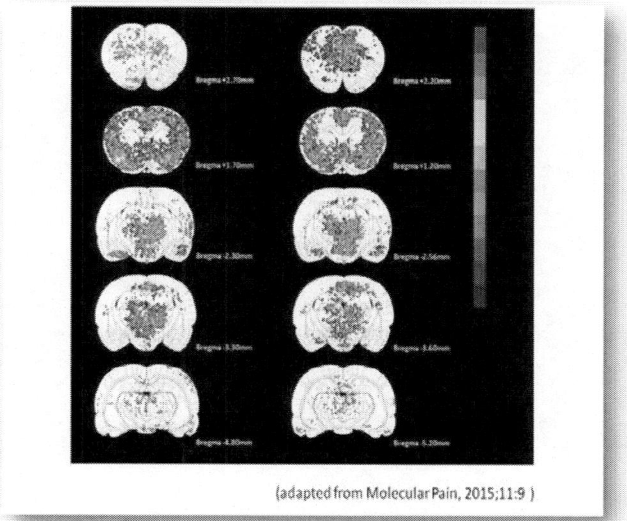

Fig. (3). Key brain regions that present significant differences in pixel counts between the CPSP and sham groups. The results were obtained by differential subtraction between the two groups. The signals in the cortex, thalamus, hypothalamus, and amygdala were significantly higher in the CPSP group than in the sham group, and the signal in the ventrobasal complex was significantly lower in the CPSP group than in the sham group. Adapted from Lu *et al.* [39]

Table 2. Key brain regions that show significant changes in [14C] signals using two different brain imaging methods.

Brain region	SPM	ROI	
	Left / Right	Left / Right	
Infralimbic cortex (IL)	P = 1.00	P = 0.02*	P = 0.00*
Prelimbic cortex (PrL)	P = 1.00	P = 0.30	P = 0.00*
Cingulate cortex area 2 (Cg2)	P = 0.28	P = 0.60	P = 1.00
Cingulate cortex area 1 (Cg1-1)	P = 1.00	P = 0.41	P = 0.00*
Cingulate cortex area 1 (Cg1-2)	P = 0.02*	P = 0.04*	P = 0.36
Secondary motor cortex (M2-1)	P = 1.00	P = 1.00	P = 0.87
Secondary motor cortex (M2-2)	P = 0.28	P = 0.04*	P = 0.00*

(Table 2) contd.....

Brain region	SPM	ROI	
	Left / Right	Left / Right	
Primary motor cortex (M1-1)	P = 1.00	P = 1.00	P = 0.86
Primary motor cortex (M1-2)	P = 0.58	P = 0.38	P = 0.88
Somatosensory cortex (S1-1)	P = 1.00	P = 0.93	P = 0.65
Somatosensory cortex (S1-2)	P = 0.53	P = 0.22	P = 0.98
Somatosensory cortex (S1-3)	P = 0.00*	P = 1.00	P = 1.00
Somatosensory cortex (S1-4)	P = 0.00*	P = 1.00	P = 1.00
Granular insular cortex (GI-1)	P = 1.00	P = 0.08	P = 0.34
Granular insular cortex (GI-2)	P = 0.82	P = 0.88	P = 0.85
Granular insular cortex (GI-3)	P = 0.00*	P = 1.00	P = 0.90
Agranular insular dorsal cortex (AID)	P = 1.00	P = 0.00*	P = 0.39
Agranular insular ventral cortex (AIV)	P = 1.00	P = 0.03*	P = 0.52
Striatum	P = 0.07	P = 1.00	P = 1.00
Hippocampus (Hippo-1)	P = 0.00*	P = 1.00	P = 1.00
Hippocampus (Hippo-2)	P = 0.00*	P = 1.00	P = 1.00
Hippocampus (Hippo-3)	P = 0.01*	P = 0.00*	P = 0.14
Mediodorsal thalamus nucleus (MD)	P = 0.00*	P = 0.54	P = 0.99
Ventral basal nucleus (VB)	P = 0.00*	P = 0.97	P = 0.00*
Ventrolateral thalamus nucleus (VL)	P = 0.00*	P = 1.00	P = 1.00
Ventromedial thalamus nucleus (VM)	P = 0.00*	P = 1.00	P = 1.00
Lateral hypothalamic area (LH)	P = 0.00*	P = 1.00	P = 1.00
Ventral medial hypothalamus nucleus (VMH)	P = 0.00*	P = 1.00	P = 1.00
Amygdala (Amygdala-1)	P = 0.00*	P = 1.00	P = 1.00
Amygdala (Amygdala-2)	P = 0.00*	P = 0.10	P = 0.01*
Periaqueductal gray (PAG)	P = 0.00*	P = 0.00*	P = 0.50

Significant increases or decreases in [14C] uptake are noted with p values, respectively, for the SPM and ROI image signals. *p < 0.05.

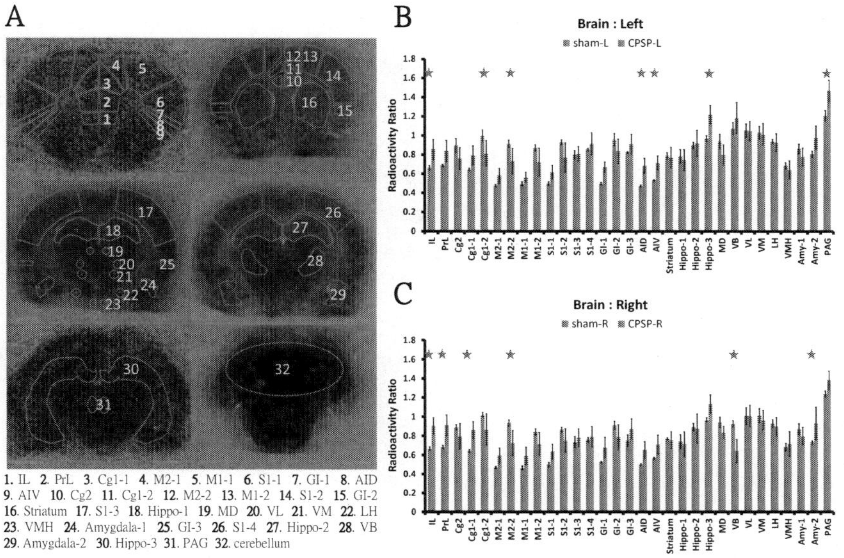

Fig. (4). Region-of-interest analysis. (A) The boundaries of the ROIs were chosen based on available anatomic atlases. (B) In the comparison of the relative ratios of the left hemisphere ROIs in the different groups, the radioactivity ratios in the infralimbic cortex, GI-3, AID, AIV, hippocampus-3, and PAG were significantly higher in the CPSP group than in the sham group, and the radioactivity ratios in the Cg1-2 and M2-2 were significantly lower in the CPSP group than in the sham group. (C) In the comparison of the relative ratios of the right hemisphere ROIs in the different groups, the radioactivity ratios in the infralimbic cortex, prelimbic cortex, Cg1-1, and amygdala-2 were significantly higher in the CPSP group than in the sham group, and the radioactivity ratios in the M2-2 and ventrobasal complex were significantly lower. (*) indicates, $p < 0.05$. Adapted from Lu *et al.* [39].

Brain activation was also subtracted between the CPSP and sham groups to reveal group differences that were analyzed by the matrix of Fisher's Z-statistic to represent differences in Pearson correlation coefficients (r). Relationships among brain areas were shown in the left and right hemispheres (Fig. **5A**, **5B**). In the left hemisphere, 114 significant correlations were found in the Pearson correlation comparisons (24.7%), including 84 positive correlations (73.7%) and 30 negative correlations (26.3%; (Fig. **5A**)). In the right hemisphere, 140 significant correlations were found in the Pearson correlation comparisons, including 104 positive correlations (74.3%) and 36 negative correlations (25.7%; (Fig. **5B**)). Therefore, the patterns of brain activation were similar between the right and left hemispheres. The left hemisphere did not present a positive correlation between the mPFC (*i.e.*, infralimbic cortex, prelimbic cortex, and Cg1) and amygdala (Fig.

5C), whereas the right hemisphere presented a positive correlation between the mPFC and amygdala. Moreover, the mPFC-amygdala pathway was shown to be connected to the PAG, thalamus, and hypothalamus (Fig. **5D**). In the left hemisphere, the prelimbic cortex and Cg1 had lower correlations with the ventromedial, ventrolateral, and mediodorsal thalamus (Fig. **5E**).

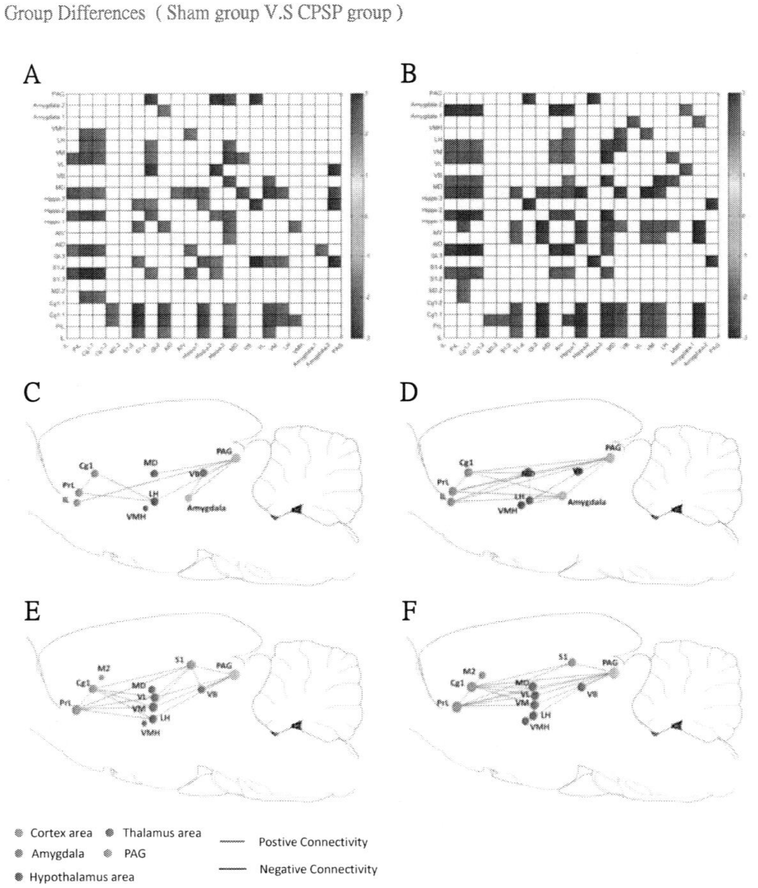

Fig. (5). Differences in inter-regional correlations of regional cerebral blood flow of neural substrates in the CPSP and sham groups. (A, B) Left and right brain connectivity. The matrix of Fisher's Z-statistic presents differences in Pearson correlation coefficients (*r*) between the CPSP and sham groups. Positive Z values indicate a greater *r* in the CPSP group, and negative Z values indicate a smaller *r*. (C-F) Inter-regional correlation of neural substrates. The ROIs are represented by nodes, and significant correlations between different ROIs are represented by different line colors. The red lines denote significant positive correlations, and the blue lines denote significant negative correlations. Adapted from Lu *et al.* [39]

However, the right hemisphere showed complex connections among many brain areas, including the spinothalamocortical and medial thalamus-anterior cingulate cortex (MT-ACC) pathways. The Cg1 and prelimbic cortex of the right hemisphere appeared to have higher correlations with the thalamus (*e.g.*, mediodorsal, ventrolateral, and ventromedial), hypothalamus (*e.g.*, lateral and ventromedial), S1, and PAG (Fig. **5F**).

Altogether, the [^{14}C] IAP assessments indicated that CPSP was associated with higher activation in the mPFC, anterior cingulate cortex, thalamus, hypothalamus, amygdala, and PAG. The inter-regional analysis of correlations indicated that the spinothalamocortical, MT-ACC, and mPFC-amygdala pathways exhibited higher activation in CPSP.

4. NEURAL CORRELATIONS AND FUNCTIONAL NETWORKS IN THE BRAIN

Previous hypotheses of pain circuitry in CPSP suggested that lesions or dysfunction of neural substrates in the spinothalamocortical pathway induce pain through impairments in the inhibition of lateral thalamus to medial thalamus connections, thus eliciting thalamic hyperactivity, thermal hyperalgesia, and mechanical allodynia [43]. Clinical human studies [31] and animal studies [41, 42] reported that the cortical pain matrix (*e.g.*, contralateral somatosensory cortex and bilateral mid- and posterior insula, anterior insula, and posterior cingulate cortex) mediates pain processing in patients with CPSP. Therefore, conventional viewpoints of pain circuitry in CPSP emphasize the involvement of the MT-ACC and spinothalamocortical pathways and pain matrix, including the somatosensory cortex, insula, and cingulate cortex (Fig. **6A**).

Our recent [^{14}C] IAP study showed complex connections between neural substrates of CPSP, with major involvement of the spinothalamocortical, MT-ACC, and mPFC-amygdala pathways [44]. The neural correlations and functional networks of CPSP are obviously different from previous reports, which we refer to as the neural correlation hypothesis [44]. CPSP may be governed by multiple pathophysiological mechanisms. For example, damage to the ventrobasal complex in the thalamus is caused by thalamic lesions and stroke hemorrhage. Thus, the ventrobasal complex cannot inhibit the information from the lateral thalamus to medial thalamus. Disinhibition of the lateral thalamus to medial thalamus connection leads to activation of the anterior cingulate cortex (a subarea of the pain matrix), resulting in CPSP symptoms (*e.g.*, thermal hyperalgesia and mechanical allodynia). Other neural substrates, including the mPFC-amygdala pathway, PAG, and hypothalamus, also become highly active, which may underlie other pathophysiological changes (Fig. **6A**).

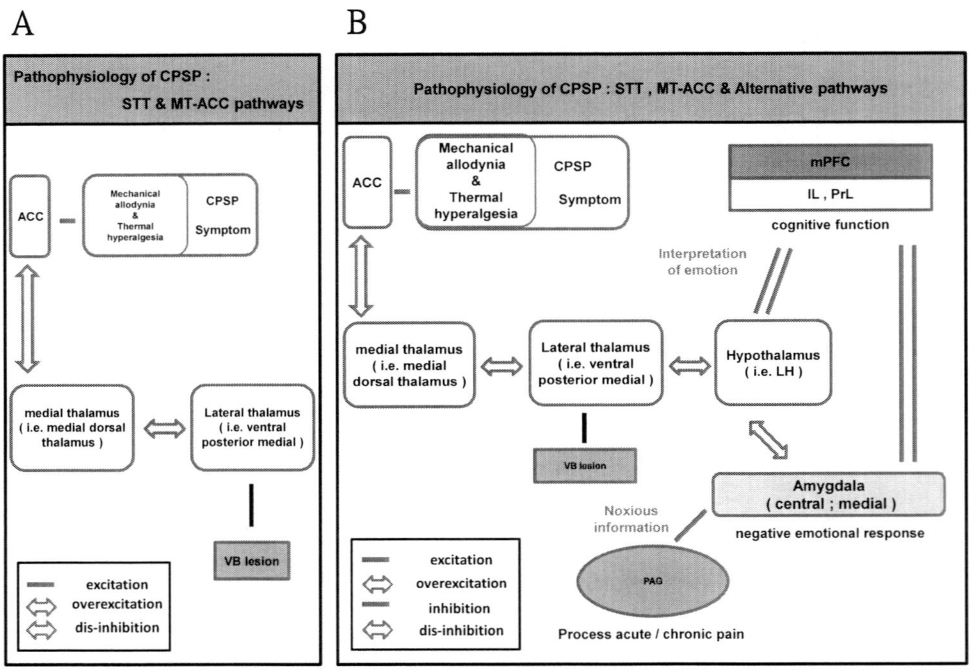

Fig. (6). Neural network hypothesis related to an animal model of CPSP. (A) Pathophysiological mechanisms in the MT-ACC pathway and STT are triggered to disinhibit the projection from the lateral thalamus and insula to medial thalamus, resulting in mechanical and thermal hyperalgesia. (B) The mPFC plays an executive function role in interactions with the amygdala, which responds to negative emotional information. The mPFC inhibits activation of the amygdala, and negative information in the amygdala is conveyed to the mPFC. The mPFC then interprets the emotional information properly. Nociceptive information from the amygdala is transmitted to the PAG to process acute and chronic pain to induce antinociception. Adapted from Lu *et al.* [39]

Subareas of the mPFC, such as the prelimbic cortex and infralimbic cortex, play a role in interpreting negative emotional responses of the central and medial amygdala, which mediate negative emotion and pain processing. Nociceptive and pain information from the amygdala is conveyed to the PAG for processing acute and spontaneous pain (Fig. **6B**).

Our proposed neural correlation hypothesis for CPSP is an extension of the classic pathophysiological viewpoint of CPSP that involves the spinothalamocortical and MT-ACC pathways and pain matrix. The mPFC-amygdala pathway, PAG, and hypothalamus are also involved in the symptoms of CPSP. Therefore, when CPSP is induced, patients present CPSP symptoms together with other symptoms, including possible motor dysfunction, depression [9, 10], anxiety [11], and cognitive dysfunction [12].

The neural correlation hypothesis of CPSP might have implications for clinical interventions and the development of novel pharmacological or non-pharmacological treatments. Such new treatments might focus on the involvement and function of different neural substrates of CPSP. For example, activation of spinothalamocortical neural circuitries and the MT-ACC pathway may be reduced to provide antinociception, and the mPFC and amygdala could become hypoactive to reduce depression and anxiety. Reduction of the activity of the PAG and hypothalamus might also result in antinociception. The distinct symptoms of CPSP may be reduced using different approaches, regardless of whether such approaches are pharmacological or non-pharmacological. Our studies of the alterations that occur in the activation of different brain areas and circuits in CPSP may provide new insights into the extensive pathophysiological mechanisms that underlie the multiple aspects of CPSP symptoms.

CONCLUSION

Three hypotheses of CPSP involve central disinhibition, central imbalance, and central sensitization. These three hypotheses do not conflict with each other, and each one can explain different aspects of the emergence and manifestation of CPSP. Based on previous studies, the central disinhibition hypothesis is often used to explain how CPSP symptoms are produced. The pain matrix and spinothalamocortical pathway have been shown to mediate CPSP in both human and animal studies. The neural correlation hypothesis of CPSP proposes that the mPFC-amygdala pathway, hypothalamus, PAG, and spinothalamocortical pathway interact with each other, resulting in CPSP symptoms. In addition to CPSP symptoms, depression, anxiety, and motor and cognitive dysfunction may be controlled by the mPFC-amygdala pathway, hypothalamus, and PAG. Our [^{14}C] IAP findings provide insights that might be applied for the development of pharmacological and non-pharmacological interventions for CPSP.

CONFLICT OF INTEREST

The authors confirm that they have no conflict of interest to declare for this publication.

ACKNOWLEDGEMENTS

This work was supported by grants from the Ministry of Science and Technology (MOST 102-2320-B-001-026-MY3 to Dr. B.C. Shyu) and National Research Council of the Republic of China (NSC 102-2410-H-431-005-MY3 to Dr. A.C.W. Huang).

REFERENCES

[1] Merskey H, Bogduk N. Classification of chronic pain: descriptions of chronic pain syndromes and definitions of pain terms. Seattle 1994.

[2] Roosink M, Geurts AC, Ijzerman MJ. Defining post-stroke pain: diagnostic challenges. Lancet Neurol 2010; 9(4): 344-5.
[http://dx.doi.org/10.1016/S1474-4422(10)70072-7] [PMID: 20298959]

[3] Kumar B, Kalita J, Kumar G, Misra UK. Central poststroke pain: a review of pathophysiology and treatment. Anesth Analg 2009; 108(5): 1645-57.
[http://dx.doi.org/10.1213/ane.0b013e31819d644c] [PMID: 19372350]

[4] Kerstman E, Ahn S, Battu S, Tariq S, Grabois M. Neuropathic pain. Handb Clin Neurol 2013; 110: 175-87.
[http://dx.doi.org/10.1016/B978-0-444-52901-5.00015-0] [PMID: 23312640]

[5] Kumar G, Soni CR. Central post-stroke pain: current evidence. J Neurol Sci 2009; 284(1-2): 10-7.
[http://dx.doi.org/10.1016/j.jns.2009.04.030] [PMID: 19419737]

[6] Klit H, Finnerup NB, Jensen TS. Central post-stroke pain: clinical characteristics, pathophysiology, and management. Lancet Neurol 2009; 8(9): 857-68.
[http://dx.doi.org/10.1016/S1474-4422(09)70176-0] [PMID: 19679277]

[7] Misra UK, Kalita J, Kumar B. A study of clinical, magnetic resonance imaging, and somatosensory-

evoked potential in central post-stroke pain. J Pain 2008; 9(12): 1116-22. [http://dx.doi.org/10.1016/j.jpain.2008.06.013] [PMID: 18848810]

[8] Edwards CL, Sudhakar S, Scales MT, Applegate KL, Webster W, Dunn RH. Electromyographic (EMG) biofeedback in the comprehensive treatment of central pain and ataxic tremor following thalamic stroke. Appl Psychophysiol Biofeedback 2000; 25(4): 229-40. [http://dx.doi.org/10.1023/A:1026406921765] [PMID: 11218924]

[9] Kim JS, Choi-Kwon S. Poststroke depression and emotional incontinence: correlation with lesion location. Neurology 2000; 54(9): 1805-10. [http://dx.doi.org/10.1212/WNL.54.9.1805] [PMID: 10802788]

[10] MacHale SM, O'Rourke SJ, Wardlaw JM, Dennis MS. Depression and its relation to lesion location after stroke. J Neurol Neurosurg Psychiatry 1998; 64(3): 371-4. [http://dx.doi.org/10.1136/jnnp.64.3.371] [PMID: 9527152]

[11] Murakami T, Hama S, Yamashita H, *et al.* Neuroanatomic pathways associated with poststroke affective and apathetic depression. Am J Geriatr Psychiatry 2013; 21(9): 840-7. [http://dx.doi.org/10.1016/j.jagp.2013.01.057] [PMID: 23567364]

[12] Chabriat H, Pappata S, Levasseur M, Fiorelli M, Tran Dinh S, Baron JC. Cortical metabolism in posterolateral thalamic stroke: PET study. Acta Neurol Scand 1992; 86(3): 285-90. [http://dx.doi.org/10.1111/j.1600-0404.1992.tb05087.x] [PMID: 1414249]

[13] Exner C, Weniger G, Irle E. Implicit and explicit memory after focal thalamic lesions. Neurology 2001; 57(11): 2054-63. [http://dx.doi.org/10.1212/WNL.57.11.2054] [PMID: 11739825]

[14] Hankey GJ, Stewart-Wynne EG. Amnesia following thalamic hemorrhage. Another stroke syndrome. Stroke 1988; 19(6): 776-8. [http://dx.doi.org/10.1161/01.STR.19.6.776] [PMID: 3376171]

[15] Gonzales GR. Central pain: diagnosis and treatment strategies. Neurology 1995; 45(12) (Suppl. 9): S11-6. [http://dx.doi.org/10.1212/WNL.45.12_Suppl_9.S11] [PMID: 8538881]

[16] Elman I, Borsook D, Volkow ND. Pain and suicidality: insights from reward and addiction neuroscience. Prog Neurobiol 2013; 109: 1-27. [http://dx.doi.org/10.1016/j.pneurobio.2013.06.003] [PMID: 23827972]

[17] Boivie J, Leijon G, Johansson I. Central post-stroke pain--a study of the mechanisms through analyses of the sensory abnormalities. Pain 1989; 37(2): 173-85. [http://dx.doi.org/10.1016/0304-3959(89)90128-0] [PMID: 2748190]

[18] Hong JH, Bai DS, Jeong JY, *et al.* Injury of the spino-thalamo-cortical pathway is necessary for central post-stroke pain. Eur Neurol 2010; 64(3): 163-8. [http://dx.doi.org/10.1159/000319040] [PMID: 20699616]

[19] Greenspan JD, Ohara S, Sarlani E, Lenz FA. Allodynia in patients with post-stroke central pain (CPSP) studied by statistical quantitative sensory testing within individuals. Pain 2004; 109(3): 357-66. [http://dx.doi.org/10.1016/j.pain.2004.02.002] [PMID: 15157697]

[20] Hong JH, Choi BY, Chang CH, *et al.* The prevalence of central poststroke pain according to the integrity of the spino-thalamo-cortical pathway. Eur Neurol 2012; 67(1): 12-7. [http://dx.doi.org/10.1159/000333012] [PMID: 22142796]

[21] Seghier ML, Lazeyras F, Vuilleumier P, Schnider A, Carota A. Functional magnetic resonance imaging and diffusion tensor imaging in a case of central poststroke pain. J Pain 2005; 6(3): 208-12. [http://dx.doi.org/10.1016/j.jpain.2004.11.004] [PMID: 15772915]

[22] Head H, Holmes G. Sensory disturbances from cerebral lesions. Brain 1911; 34: 102-254. [http://dx.doi.org/10.1093/brain/34.2-3.102]

[23] Bromm B, Frieling A, Lankers J. Laser-evoked brain potentials in patients with dissociated loss of pain and temperature sensibility. Electroencephalogr Clin Neurophysiol 1991; 80(4): 284-91. [http://dx.doi.org/10.1016/0168-5597(91)90111-A] [PMID: 1713838]

[24] Berić A, Dimitrijević MR, Lindblom U. Central dysesthesia syndrome in spinal cord injury patients. Pain 1988; 34(2): 109-16. [http://dx.doi.org/10.1016/0304-3959(88)90155-8] [PMID: 3174149]

[25] Jeanmonod D, Magnin M, Morel A. Low-threshold calcium spike bursts in the human thalamus. Common physiopathology for sensory, motor and limbic positive symptoms. Brain 1996; 119(Pt 2): 363-75. [http://dx.doi.org/10.1093/brain/119.2.363] [PMID: 8800933]

[26] Lenz FA, Kwan HC, Martin R, Tasker R, Richardson RT, Dostrovsky JO. Characteristics of somatotopic organization and spontaneous neuronal activity in the region of the thalamic principal sensory nucleus in patients with spinal cord transection. J Neurophysiol 1994; 72(4): 1570-87. [PMID: 7823087]

[27] Peyron R, Garcia-Larrea L, Deiber MP, *et al.* Electrical stimulation of precentral cortical area in the treatment of central pain: electrophysiological and PET study. Pain 1995; 62(3): 275-86. [http://dx.doi.org/10.1016/0304-3959(94)00211-V] [PMID: 8657427]

[28] Rinaldi PC, Young RF, Albe-Fessard D, Chodakiewitz J. Spontaneous neuronal hyperactivity in the medial and intralaminar thalamic nuclei of patients with deafferentation pain. J Neurosurg 1991; 74(3): 415-21. [http://dx.doi.org/10.3171/jns.1991.74.3.0415] [PMID: 1993906]

[29] Pomares FB, Faillenot I, Barral FG, Peyron R. The 'where' and the 'when' of the BOLD response to pain in the insular cortex. Discussion on amplitudes and latencies. Neuroimage 2013; 64: 466-75. [http://dx.doi.org/10.1016/j.neuroimage.2012.09.038] [PMID: 23006804]

[30] Ducreux D, Attal N, Parker F, Bouhassira D. Mechanisms of central neuropathic pain: a combined psychophysical and fMRI study in syringomyelia. Brain 2006; 129(Pt 4): 963-76. [http://dx.doi.org/10.1093/brain/awl016] [PMID: 16434417]

[31] Symonds LL, Gordon NS, Bixby JC, Mande MM. Right-lateralized pain processing in the human cortex: an FMRI study. J Neurophysiol 2006; 95(6): 3823-30. [http://dx.doi.org/10.1152/jn.01162.2005] [PMID: 16554508]

[32] Craig AD, Reiman EM, Evans A, Bushnell MC. Functional imaging of an illusion of pain. Nature 1996; 384(6606): 258-60.

[http://dx.doi.org/10.1038/384258a0] [PMID: 8918874]

[33] Kassubek J, Juengling FD, Els T, *et al.* Activation of a residual cortical network during painful stimulation in long-term postanoxic vegetative state: a 15O-H2O PET study. J Neurol Sci 2003; 212(1-2): 85-91.
[http://dx.doi.org/10.1016/S0022-510X(03)00106-0] [PMID: 12810004]

[34] Kwan CL, Crawley AP, Mikulis DJ, Davis KD. An fMRI study of the anterior cingulate cortex and surrounding medial wall activations evoked by noxious cutaneous heat and cold stimuli. Pain 2000; 85(3): 359-74.
[http://dx.doi.org/10.1016/S0304-3959(99)00287-0] [PMID: 10781909]

[35] Maarrawi J, Peyron R, Mertens P, *et al.* Differential brain opioid receptor availability in central and peripheral neuropathic pain. Pain 2007; 127(1-2): 183-94.
[http://dx.doi.org/10.1016/j.pain.2006.10.013] [PMID: 17137714]

[36] Willoch F, Schindler F, Wester HJ, *et al.* Central poststroke pain and reduced opioid receptor binding within pain processing circuitries: a [11C]diprenorphine PET study. Pain 2004; 108(3): 213-20.
[http://dx.doi.org/10.1016/j.pain.2003.08.014] [PMID: 15030940]

[37] Matharu MS, Bartsch T, Ward N, Frackowiak RS, Weiner R, Goadsby PJ. Central neuromodulation in chronic migraine patients with suboccipital stimulators: a PET study. Brain 2004; 127(Pt 1): 220-30.
[http://dx.doi.org/10.1093/brain/awh022] [PMID: 14607792]

[38] Ohn SH, Chang WH, Park CH, *et al.* Neural correlates of the antinociceptive effects of repetitive transcranial magnetic stimulation on central pain after stroke. Neurorehabil Neural Repair 2012; 26(4): 344-52.
[http://dx.doi.org/10.1177/1545968311423110] [PMID: 21980153]

[39] Rainville P, Bushnell MC, Duncan GH. Representation of acute and persistent pain in the human CNS: potential implications for chemical intolerance. Ann N Y Acad Sci 2001; 933: 130-41.
[http://dx.doi.org/10.1111/j.1749-6632.2001.tb05820.x] [PMID: 12000016]

[40] Staud R, Craggs JG, Robinson ME, Perlstein WM, Price DD. Brain activity related to temporal summation of C-fiber evoked pain. Pain 2007; 129(1-2): 130-42.
[http://dx.doi.org/10.1016/j.pain.2006.10.010] [PMID: 17156923]

[41] Hess A, Sergejeva M, Budinsky L, Zeilhofer HU, Brune K. Imaging of hyperalgesia in rats by functional MRI. Eur J Pain 2007; 11(1): 109-19.
[http://dx.doi.org/10.1016/j.ejpain.2006.01.005] [PMID: 16517192]

[42] Jiang L, Ji Y, Voulalas PJ, *et al.* Motor cortex stimulation suppresses cortical responses to noxious hindpaw stimulation after spinal cord lesion in rats. Brain Stimulat 2014; 7(2): 182-9.
[http://dx.doi.org/10.1016/j.brs.2013.12.013] [PMID: 24468093]

[43] Wang Z, Bradesi S, Maarek JM, *et al.* Regional brain activation in conscious, nonrestrained rats in response to noxious visceral stimulation. Pain 2008; 138(1): 233-43.
[http://dx.doi.org/10.1016/j.pain.2008.04.018] [PMID: 18538929]

[44] Lu HC, Chang WJ, Kuan YH, Huang AC, Shyu BC. A [14C]iodoantipyrine study of inter-regional correlations of neural substrates following central post-stroke pain in rats. Mol Pain 2015; 11: 9.
[http://dx.doi.org/10.1186/s12990-015-0006-5] [PMID: 25889278]

CHAPTER 3

The Role of Psychological Factors in Cardiac and Non-Cardiac Chest Pain

Masoumali Masoumi[1], **Mozhgan Saeidi**[2] and **Saeid Komasi**[2,*]

[1] *Cardiac Surgery, Bistoon Hospital, Kermanshah, Iran*

[2] *Cardiac Rehabilitation Center, Imam Ali Hospital, Kermanshah University of Medical Sciences, Kermanshah, Iran*

Abstract: Chest pain as a common symptom in general population is considered to be the second most common cause of presentation to emergency departments of medical centers. Such pains are categorized broadly into cardiac chest pain (CCP) *vs.* non-cardiac chest pain (NCCP). In patients with cardiac diseases, the main symptoms of psychological reactions to pain include psychological stress, fear and anxiety, pain resulting from anxiety, and anxiety and depression as a result of pain. Furthermore, there is a relationship between perceived psychological factors and the psychological distress, and sustained NCCP could lead to the development of depression, stress and low mental quality of life. Controlled clinical trials on treating CCP and NCCP have shown that these relatively extensive interventions have been effective in reducing psychological distress, periods of chest pain frequency, and lowering functional problems.

Keywords: Angina pectoris, Cardiac chest pain, Cardiovascular diseases, Cognitive - behavior therapy, Non-cardiac chest pain, Psychological distress, Psychological factors, Psychotherapy.

INTRODUCTION

Since life-threatening events in patients with or without established cardiovascular diseases (CVDs) occur suddenly, chest pain experience could be horrifying for

* **Coresponding author Saeid Komasi:** Cardiac Rehabilitation Center, Imam Ali Hospital, Kermanshah University of Medical Sciences, Shahid Beheshti Boulevard, Kermanshah, Iran; E-mail:S_komasi63@yahoo.com

Puneetpal Singh (Ed.)

anyone [1]. Chest pain as a common symptom in general population is considered to be the second most common cause of presentation to emergency departments (ED) of medical clinics and hospitals [2]. In the US, six million patients present to ED annually. This imposes over eight billion US$ on healthcare system [3]. Chest pain, with a life time prevalence of 39%, affects the quality of life of suffering patient severely and results in decreased working ability, physical exercise and serious sleep problems [4 - 7]. Chest pain, especially as it may herald serious cardiac conditions like heart attack, cause nervousness and consequently lead in apparent complaining by patients [8]. Chest pain presents itself in various forms such as phrictopathic sensation, hot flashes, tingling, pressure sensation, and choking. It also varies in terms of duration and severity [9]. Such pains are categorized broadly into cardiac chest pain (CCP) *vs.* non-cardiac chest pain (NCCP).

CARDIAC CHEST PAIN (CCP)

Cardiovascular diseases (CVDs), as one of the most common conditions, are responsible for disability in 151 million patients and death in 17 million cases of the world population. Even though 14% of disabilities and 30% of mortality cases in developed countries are attributed to CVDs, about 82% of disabilities and 75% of death cases in developing countries are the result of such diseases [10]. One of the symptoms of cardiac disease is chest pain which is considered as one of the most prevalent cause of presentation of patients to cardiovascular clinics [11]. CCP are usually the result of acute coronary syndrome (ACS), myocardial infarction (MI) or ischemia, aortic dissection, pericarditis, cardiac arrhythmias, anxiety and panic attacks.

The pain of MI, myocardial ischemia, pericarditis, and greater vessels disease are considered as one of the most common causes of CCP. The pain of MI or myocardial ischemia happens when the required oxygen of the myocardium is not supplied. But infectious pericarditis pain always involves the surroundings of the pleura and cause pleuritic pain in patients. This pain aggravates with inspiration, coughing, and bodily position change. However, in patients with vascular diseases, acute aortic dissection causes a sudden, tearing, and severely distressing pain [12]. Pain is a mental phenomenon associated with unpleasant feelings and causes distress. Pain-related complaints are the most common symptoms experienced by patients [13].

Epidemiology

Annually, seven million Americans present to ED because of acute chest pain. About 15-25% of such presentations are due to CVDs [12]. The prevalence of angina pectoris increases with aging in both males and females and it is estimated that 2-4% of adult population in the Europe experience CCP [14]. According to Modi *et al.* (2015), of patients who admit in ED because of chest pain, less than 50% are discharged in a short time and only 7.2% of those who are admitted have CVDs [15]. In another study, it has been reported that in 9.6% of the cases, the cause of chest pain is CADs [16].

Etiology

CCP is the result of decreased blood supply by coronary arteries or increased demand for oxygen by the myocardium [17]. The most common cause of acute chest pain in patients with CVDs is MI or myocardial ischemia and happens when enough oxygen is not supplied to the heart [12]. This pain which can be continuous or intermittent is known as angina pectoris. Angina can be affected by factors other than cardiac diseases such as psychological factors.

Cardiac Chest Pain and Mechanism of Pain

Chest pain, while having many etiologies, is generally considered to be most lethal when related to a cardiac cause [18]. Cardiac chest pain or angina pectoris can be either acute or chronic and usually is a result of imbalance between myocardial oxygen supply and myocardial oxygen demand. Atheroma formation and atherosclerotic plaques seem to affect coronary flow, given that multivessel flow-limiting obstructions are observed in patients with chronic coronary syndrome. In addition, morphological changes of diseased arteries related to significant atherosclerosis, such as vascular remodeling may also result in stable angina or claudication [19].

Although, angina pectoris has a variety of physiological correlates, including the type of triggering activity, the severity of ischemia or ventricular dysfunction, adenosine release, endogenous opiate response, and pain threshold, a variety of psychological characteristics have also been found to be associated with it. The patients highly report depression, state anxiety, trait anxiety compared with patients with history of angina [20]. Emotional stress provokes angina by increasing the myocardial oxygen consumption above a critical level and it may be associated with increased venous tone which might lead to an increase in central venous pressure and ventricular volume [21]. Although, emotional stress provoked a transient, relative decrease in myocardial oxygen delivery [21], the positive psychological state of an individual can modulate cardiac nociception *via* pathways involving the amygdala [22].

Myocardial Ischemia Syndrome

The pathophysiological events that occur at the coronary atherosclerotic plaque have been of great interest for the past few decades. As classically described in literatures, fatty plaque progressively builds up to obstructive atherosclerotic plaque, causing myocardial ischemia and angina. Although at any stage of this progression, plaque rupture, fissure, or erosion may lead to thrombotic occlusion and precipitate illness, obstructive plaque is only one of the manifestations of atherosclerotic disease. Indeed, a number of alternative atherosclerotic mechanisms, including "spontaneous" thrombosis, coronary vasospasm, inflammation, microvascular dysfunction, endothelial dysfunction, and angiogenesis, have been shown to be capable of precipitating myocardial ischemia and angina [23].

Ischemic heart disease can occur in the presence or absence of obstructive coronary artery disease and that atherosclerosis is just one element in a complex multifactorial pathophysiological process that includes inflammation, endothelial dysfunction, microvascular coronary dysfunction, thrombosis, and angiogenesis. Furthermore, the high recurrence rates underscore the fact that removing stenosis in patients with stable Ischemic heart disease does not address the underlying pathological mechanisms that lead to the progression of nonculprit lesions. The role of inflammation is confirmed as a important part of the pathological process. Monocytederived macrophages and T lymphocytes produce and secrete mediator molecules (enzymes, cytokines, chemokines, growth factors, and disintegrins), which activate endothelial cells, increase vasoreactivity, and cause proliferation of smooth muscle cells and lesion progression. Endothelial dysfunction through regulation of vascular tone, platelet activity, leukocyte adhesion, and thrombosis, is a predictor of ischemic heart disease in patients [23]. Microvascular coronary dysfunction is the predominant etiological mechanism of ischemia in approximately 50% of patients with the persistent chest pain [24]. In addition, coronary thrombi were shown to overlay the intima of a coronary vessel independently of plaque type and severity. Thus, it can be said that obstructive atherosclerosis is neither a sufficient nor a necessary cause for Ischemic heart disease and chest pain but just one component of a complex pathophysiological process [23].

Myocardial Ischemia and Mechanism of Pain

The experience of pain related to cardiac ischemia is a complex issue and is likely influenced by a number of factors. Individuals with myocardial ischemia may or may not experience pain during such episodes, or they may experience pain during some ischemic episodes and not others. Some people may complain of chest pain that is not cardiac related, but also have pain resulting from myocardial ischemia. According to recent reports, pain is a biopsychosocial phenomenon, that an interaction of biological, psychological, and social factors may explain angina and the variability in symptoms that accompany it (Fig. **1**). However, the true distinction between the biological *versus* psychological *versus* social aspects of illness are dependent on the way they are measured rather than on the mechanism of action [25].

Biological factors included mechanical and chemical factors, comorbid conditions, sex and racial differences. Painful sensations may be due to mechanical factors such as spasm or distention of cardiac vessels. The lesions present with arteriosclerosis interfere with increases in blood flow necessary to meet increased cardiac demand, which may lead to pain. Mechanical distension of the coronary artery wall may activate sensory receptors at the periarterial level and cause pain. Increased lactic acid, release of potassium ions, and production of kinins and other pain-producing substances in myocardial ischemia are as chemical factors affecting the pain. Furthermore, patients with comorbidities such as diabetes, hypertension, kidney disease, and peripheral vascular disease, African Americans compared with Caucasians, and females compared with males experience pain in different ways [25].

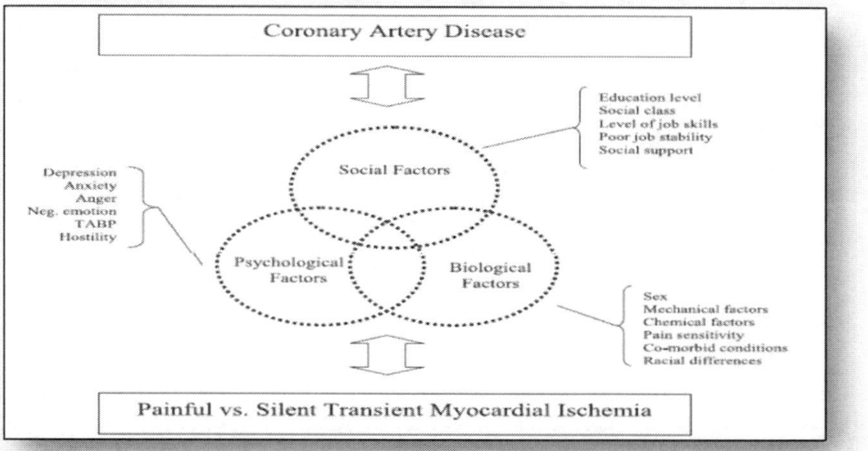

Fig. (1). An interactive model of pain and myocardial ischemia (Adapted from Hofkamp *et al.* 2007).

Psychological factors, including depression, stress, anxiety, anger, quality of life, negative emotion/distress, personality, and beliefs about angina, and social factors such as social support also are effect in experienced angina [25 - 28]. Anxiety and stress may exacerbate pain through increased heart rate and blood pressure, centrally-mediated neurogenic peripheral vasoconstriction, and catecholamine release [28]. Anxiety symptoms also associated with depression.

Depression not only is associated with cardiovascular risk factors including smoking, sedentary lifestyle, obesity, diabetes, and hypertension, but it have an independent effect on cardiac outcomes after adjustment for these factors [29]. Exercise-induced ST segment depression is the single most significant variable in relation to the amount of ischemic myocardium [30]. So, angina may be affected by depression.

Dissecan Aortic Aneurysm and Mechanisms of Pain

The term *aortic aneurysm* refers to a pathologic segment of aortic dilation that has a propensity to expand and rupture. Aortic aneurysms are either fusiform or saccular. Fusiform aneurysms are most common and are characterized by a general symmetric dilation with a fairlyuniform shape involving the entire aortic wall circumference. Saccular aneurysms exhibit localized dilation involving only a portion of the aortic wall circumference, appearing as a focal outpouching. These lesions represent true aneurysms in that the aortic wall is intact but dilated, involving all layers of aortic structure. In contrast, pseudoaneurysms (false aneurysms) represent lesions in which there has been bleeding through the aortic wall, resulting in a contained periaortic hematoma in continuity with the aortic lumen. These lesions may result from trauma or from contained rupture of an aortic aneurysm, dissection, or penetrating ulcer [31].

Acute aortic dissection is the most common catastrophic event affecting the aorta, with an estimated annual incidence of approximately 5 to 30 per million. There are two main hypotheses for acute aortic dissection. The first is that an aortic dissection may be related to a primary tear in the aortic intima, with blood from the aortic lumen penetrating into the diseased media, leading to dissection and creating the true and false lumen. The second main hypothesis is that a primary rupture of the vasa vasorum leads to hemorrhage in the aortic wall, with subsequent intimal disruption, creating the intimal tear and aortic dissection. The pressure of the pulsatile blood within the aortic wall after dissection leads to extension of the dissection [31].

The most serious complications of aortic aneurysms are rupture and dissection [31]. Aortic rupture is that affected by a history of hypertension [32], leads to sudden severe chest or back pain. Persistent chest pain may occur because of a direct mass effect from the aortic aneurysm, with compression of the intrathoracic structures or erosion into adjacent bones. Furthermore, acute aortic expansion, contained rupture, and pseudoaneurysm can cause severe chest pain [31].

Endothelial Dysfunction and the Impact of Psychological Factors

The vascular endothelium secretes factors that not only adapt blood vessel tone, but also contribute in the development and progression of atherosclerosis through their effects on platelet adhesion and aggregation, cell proliferation, and thrombogenicity. Coronary endothelial dysfunction in the coronary microcirculation, mainly the arterioles is said to be the trigger for pathogenesis of ischemic heart disease. Intact endothelium has a vital role in the regulation of vascular tone by releasing nitric oxide and thus matching myocardial perfusion with oxygen consumption. Furthermore, myocardial ischemia may occur with impaired endothelium-dependent coronary flow reserve of the coronary epicardial and microcirculation, supporting a role for the coronary epicardial and microcirculation endothelium in regulating myocardial perfusion [24].

Hemodynamic forces (wail shear and turbulence) are thought to play the initiating role in causing endothelial damage. These forces are more common at the arterial branches and bifurcations where atherosclerotic plaques usually develop. Endothelial injury is followed by the adherence of platelets, release of platelet-derived growth factor, the migration of monocytes into the intima, and migration and proliferation of smooth muscle from the media. These result in the production of an atherosclerotic plaque. Repeated episodes of injury result in progressive narrowing of the vascular lumen by a vicious cycle of flow disturbance, endothelial injury, and plaque growth [33].

Psychological factors also are effective in the development of endothelial dysfunction and chest pain. The presence of emotional distress, other than clinical levels of depression and anxiety, has been documented as a common comorbidity found in all types of chest pain [25]. Furthermore, psychological stress causes epicardial coronary and microvascular vasoconstriction in patients with endothelial dysfunction. Psychological stress unleashes an increase in heart rate and in blood pressure, which are measured through stimulation of adrenergic sympathetic activity. In healthy individuals, the integer endothelium promotes a compensatory vasodilator response to sympathetic stimulus. In carriers of coronary arterial disease, whose physiopathologic basis is the endothelial dysfunction, this compensatory mechanism is damaged, which leads to a significant coronary vasoconstriction and to alterations in the myocardial offer and demand of oxygen. An inappropriate response may cause ventricular contraction dysfunction, myocardial ischemia or cardiac rhythm disorders. Due to physiopathologic differences between physical, pharmacological and psychological stress, individual variations in the response to each stimulus are expected [34]. However, several studies indicate that treatment of emotional distress with cognitive-behavioral therapy reduces angina symptoms [35, 36].

Psychological Etiology

Psychological and psychiatric factors play major role in chest pain and its severity perception [37]. Based on the report by Bekkouche *et al.* (2013), emotional-cognitive as well as cognitive-interpersonal factors are affective in exercise-induced angina in patients with ischemic heart disease (IHD) [38]. Of these factors, stress, depression, anxiety, anger, and hostility can be mentioned. Stress, as one of the affective psychological factors on the health, can cause endothelial dysfunction in patients with angina. This disturbance can have relationship with symptom aggravation [39]. Daily stress has relationship with cardiac symptoms, especially angina pectoris [40]. Psychological stressors, in particular mental stress, are considered triggers for cardiac ischemic periods and CCP and have important role in angina pectoris frequency [41]. Apart from stress, depression and anxiety are the most common psychiatric disorders that can have role in development of angina pectoris among cardiac patients [11, 20, 42, 43]. Garganeeva *et al.* (2014) stated that depression in cardiac patients is associated with the risk of poor prognosis, simultaneous injuries, psychosocial stress, poorer quality of life, and more severe angina [44]. Depression and anxiety are associated with poor prognosis of coronary artery disease (CAD) and recurrent cardiac events. Apart from this, these duos also increase the chance of chest pain during anger episodes [45]. It should be noted that anger and hostility are influential factors on CCP. The results of several studies show that increased anger and hostility scores in cardiac patients can result in more frequent and more severe episodes of chest pain [46 - 48]. In total, psychological factors especially depression, anxiety, anger and hostility can cause development of cardiac condition [49 - 51], and consequently happening and aggravation of chest pain. The role of these psychological factors in development of cardiac conditions is so prominent that 33.7% of males and 38.2% of females mention these factors as the main cause of their disease [52]. It is obvious that this condition can have role in improvement of symptoms, especially chest pain.

Cardiac patients mention psychological factors like Stress, anxiety, depression and grief while discussing the etiology of their disease after behavioral factors [53]. On the other hand, several studies show that causal beliefs of patients about cardiac disease are strongly associated with risk factors [54 - 56]. When perceived and actual risk factors are compared, the significant attention is paid to psychological risk factors by patients. It makes the importance of psychological risk factors in development of CVDs and their negative consequences on the disease outcomes obvious. According to Channer *et al.* (1988), those with CVDs who have psychiatric disorders experience more severe angina compared to other patients [57]. Therefore, it seems that the risk factors, indirectly and possibly by affecting the patient's physiological status, can stabilize and intensify pain following cardiac event.

CCP Outcomes and Psychological Distress

Tachycardia/palpitation and CCP are associated with situations such as inappropriate conflict resolution, aggression or passive conflict, insecurity and instability in relationships, a sense of being worse than spouse and future financial problems [58]. The reason behind these negative outcomes can be patients' cognitions and understanding of the pain phenomenon. For example, patients who are more optimistic report less severe physical symptoms and pain [59]. Also, extroverted patients, in comparison to introverted patients, exhibit less unpleasant reactions to sadness and have significantly lower heart rate reaction to sadness and pain symptoms [60]. Etherton *et al.* (2014) stated that patients' perception can be affected by their mood and negative perception can predict their worse situation [61]. Schroeder *et al.* (2012) stated that there is relationship between perceptional-cognitional factors and pain severity in patients with CCP [62]. In fact, the way that cardiac disease and related pain is perceived increases pain severity and can have personal, social, occupational, and psychological outcomes in patients. Patients with CVDs suffering from chest pain typically leave more work days and experience more impaired social function [5]. They are seriously facing with impaired quality of life and develop depression [63]. In patients with stable angina, one episode of angina per week or fewer attacks is associated with increasing physical limitations and poorer quality of life [64]. Patients with CCP, especially when they are depressed, present to physicians more because of cardiac symptoms [65] and lose more days in occupational and personal life domains.

In patients with cardiac conditions, although chest pain is associated with anxiety, depression and overall distress [66], psychological stress is quite common [13]. Even though such patients experience anxiety and depression [5], perceived stress and anger, do not face problems as much as patients with non-cardiac chest pain (NCCP) [67]. In patients with cardiac diseases, the main symptoms of psychological reactions to pain include psychological stress, fear and anxiety, pain resulting from anxiety, and anxiety and depression as a result of pain [13]. Any of these factors can arise as the outcome of pain with particular mechanism. For instance, increasing anxiety, less physical activity and pain severity are under the influence of heart stress reaction in patients with CVDs [68]. This group of patients, especially those who have received invasive treatments such as coronary artery bypass graft (CABG), experience more anxiety, which can result in increased pain perception [69]. On the other hand, increased perception of pain can be the result of anxiety and fear resulted by mental grading of pain by patients [60]. This state along with angina attacks results in decreased quality of life in psychological, physical, social domains and quality of life in general and inappropriate control of this pain can have negative effects on quality of life [70]. In fact, CCP is a negative predictor of quality of life in cardiac patients [64], in a way that one-third of patients with CVDs complain of angina after successful angioplasty and this pain causes severe limitation in their quality of life [71].

CCP and Psychotherapy

Since psychological factors are effective in establishment and aggravation of CCP, it has been suggested to employ psychological interventions in order to decrease negative outcomes of pain. Psychological interventions can decrease the rate of angina pectoris in short term [72]. Psychological treatment and evaluation can help patients with CCP *via* effect on development and progression of the disease. Such psychological interventions can expand and promote behavioral changes and increase treatment adherence by patients [1]. These interventions are broad and include cognitive-behavioral therapy (CBT) methods and other methods such as stress control and management strategies, pain confrontation strategies, emotion regulation strategies, relaxation training, meditation, hypnotherapy, music therapy, self-management designs, and social support.

The methods based on stress reduction and pain confrontation strategies have gained attention, as one of the primary treatment methods, in recent years. Balgard *et al.* (2014) stated that the intervention of stress control in cardiac patients resulted in decreased blood pressure, heart rate, serum cholesterol and increased heart activity and resultant pain sensitivity in patients with CVDs [73]. Also, since patients with cardiac problems who have fear and anxiety are generally under the dominance of strong interests for self-blame and experiencing feeling of guilt and high levels of internal tension, it seems that educating pain confrontation strategies is an effective approach to decrease psychological symptoms and pain. These strategies are considered psychotherapy methods employed to decrease aggressive tendencies and internal tensions in such patients. These strategies are real effort to change perception and thinking method regarding pain [13].

In addition, since it has been advised to pay attention to emotional irregularities in patients with chronic pain [74], a study investigated the effect of emotional regulation strategies on decreases in pain in such patients. According to the results of this study, emotional regulation strategies resulted in decreased verbal and non-verbal indices of pain. Conscious use of emotional regulation strategies during painful activities adjusted pain-related statements both cognitive and automatically [75].

Relaxation training is one of the cognitive-behavioral therapy (CBT) methods which can create physiologic effects contrary to anxiety (slow heart rate, increased peripheral vascular circulation and neuromuscular stability). Relaxation training decreases the occurrence of angina pectoris, cardiac arrhythmias and ischemia and promotes return to occupational activities and also decreases future cardiac events and death [76]. Relaxation training in cardiac patients, in particular after coronary artery bypass graft (CABG), increases the overall well-being and decreases pain [77]. Also, community-based meditation results in better quality of life, decreased psychological distress, increased tolerability, decreased body mass index and blood pressure [78] and probably decreased pain symptoms in patients with CVDs.

Hypnotherapy and music therapy can also be effective. Zamuner *et al.* (2015) in their study about the effect of hypnotherapy on women with cardiac diseases concluded that this therapeutic method for 16 weeks resulted in improved exercise capacity, decreased cardiac sympathetic modulation, improved automatic match between the heart and orthostatic stimuli, improved quality of life and decreased pain symptoms [79]. Music therapy also significantly decreases stress-related hormones, heart rate, systolic and diastolic blood pressures, and finally pain in patients who have experienced MI [69].

In addition to the above mentioned methods, there are other methods in which role of patients and their supportive system becomes important. One of these is self-management of angina, which is developed for those who are suffering from angina pectoris. This method can be significantly influential in decreasing anxiety and improving perceived quality of life [71]. Plus pain self-management, social support is also important; the results of study by Roberts *et al.* (2015) show that social support causes decrease in blood pressure and heart rate, cortisol reactivity, tension and finally CCP [80].

The Indications for Psychotherapy and Hypnotherapy

Although a cardiac event with any origin usually comes with a lot of stress and distress, psychotherapy delivered to patients is inevitable and necessary at each stage of the disease. Psychological assessment of patients by short and appropriate tools can be effective in providing timely services. In the first step, patient's causal beliefs should be monitored. Because of inconsistency between the perceived and real risk factors can affect patient understanding, increase anxiety, and can pave the way for development of psychological disorders like depression [81]. According to the results of a recent study, cardiac patients with physiological or psychological perceived risk factor highly experience depression with compared to patients with behavioral perceived risk factor [81]. Furthermore, beliefs about angina are significantly associated with functional and psychological status. Obtained results by Furze *et al.* (2005) indicate patients with more misconceived or maladaptive beliefs were more anxious and physically limited than were others with fewer such beliefs. In addition, change in angina beliefs over 1 year is the most significant predictor for physical functioning at follow-up

[27]. So, psychotherapy, especially cognitive therapy, is preferred to hypnotherapy.

NON-CARDIAC CHEST PAIN (NCCP)

NCCP is defined as pain similar to angina but without any evidence indicating CAD. This pain manifests itself with various symptoms. NCCP may be felt in chest, involve the anterior wall of the chest or may be felt originating from chest area. NCCP can be manifested with patterns similar to CAD and its duration varies from minutes to hours [82]. Based on different studies, in 60-90% of presentations to ED because of chest pain, there is no evidence of cardiac-origin pain [3] and generally there is no history of cardiac disease in more than 50% of such patients [83]. However, these patients present frequently to medical centers seeking for medical attention. Resultant medical and diagnostic evaluations cost so much for healthcare systems [84].

Epidemiology

In general, according to the reports, the prevalence of NCCP was reported as 33 percent, of which, almost 23 percent of patients visit physician for these symptoms [85]. Although 70 million people (equivalent to 23 percent of US population) have reported complaints on NCCP, it is merely in 15-25 percent of the cases that pain has cardiac origin [12]. This amount might differ in various places as the demographic studies in various countries have reported following rates: Australia: 33 percent [4], China: 21 percent [86], Argentina: 24 percent [87] and Spain: 8-28 percent [88].

Etiology

On the topic of the etiology and continuity of NCCP, a multi-factorial state with different physiological and psychological factors could be discussed [9]. The physiological factors include pulmonary aspects (such as respiratory infections), musculoskeletal complications (such as thoracic wall spasm) and problems caused by gastritis (reflux or esophageal disorders) [89]. Nevertheless, no apparent physical cause could be confirmed in almost 50 to 66 percent of patients [90, 91]. But psychological [82] and psychiatric [92] factors are involved.

Psychological Etiology

The role of psychological factors in the appearance and continuity of NCCP is so important that it has been shown that patients with psychiatric problems with hospitalization records are significantly more in risk of mortality and pre-term cardiovascular complications compared to patients without such records [93]. The results of studies carried out by Jerlock *et al.* (2007) showed that health-related life style of patients with NCCP is poorer compared with general population. These patients show more concern on work stress, experience more perceived stress at home, have more problems in sleeping and experience more frequent negative events in life [90]. Although these patients use cognitive coping strategies for controlling and managing stress, their emotional reaction to stress intensifies or increases the frequency of their chest pain. The irrational beliefs in this group of patients which are effective in their emotional reactions are among these factors that give way to pain intensity in such a way that patients with more irrational beliefs report higher intensity of pain [94].

So far, different studies [85, 95] have shown the relationship between psychological disorders and the poor future consequences in patients with NCCP complaints. The poor psychological consequences in this group of patients include higher rates of mental disorders [92, 96] especially panic attacks, anxiety and depression [45, 97 - 99]. The results of studies conducted by White *et al.* (2008) reported 41 percent prevalence of any types of anxiety disorders, 12 percent panic attacks, 16 percent social phobia, 13 percent generalized anxiety disorder (GAD), 14 percent specific phobia and 8 percent depression among patients with NCCP [92]. Another study reported the prevalence of panic attacks in 15 percent of cases, any anxiety disorders in 32 percent, major depression in 5 percent, any somatoforms in 13 percent, drug abuse in 4 percent and psychiatric disorders in 38 percent of cases [6].

High frequency of anxiety disorders in NCCP shows that anxiety can trigger NCCP, intensify it or stabilize it [100, 101]. Therefore, anxiety disorders perhaps play an important role in the manifestation of NCCP symptoms [102]. Depression is also considered as one of the most important psychological disorder that plays role both in the appearance and continuity of NCCP [103]. In the meantime, in addition to anxiety or depression, alexithymia [104] and more negative emotions such as emotional/verbal and physical abuses [105] are reported to be involved in higher rate of NCCP appearance [106] and this psychological condition might remain undiagnosed in up to 83 percent of cases [107].

Differential Diagnosis

According to the relevant literature, gastroesophageal reflux disorders (GERD), musculoskeletal chest wall pain, oesophageal abnormalities, pulmonary disorders, and psychological disorders are the major causes of NCCP [108]. In patients with NCCP, thorough clinical evaluation of the patient's history, symptoms, and clinical findings can indicate the most appropriate diagnostic tests. For instance, GERD is more likely with a positive response to a proton pump inhibitor test. So, treatment response to high-dose proton pump inhibitor treatment provides important information regarding GERD, and should be considered early. GERD diagnosis is also more likely with typical GERD symptoms than atypical GERD symptoms [3]. On other hand, common causes of musculoskeletal chest wall pain included isolated musculoskeletal chest wall pain (costochondritis, lower rib pain syndrome, sternalis syndrome, thoracic costovertebral joint dysfunction), rheumatic causes (fibromyalgia, rheumatoid arthritis, axial spondyloarthropathy, psoriatic arthritis), and non-rheumatic systemic causes (osteoporotic fracture, neoplasm with pathological fracture or bone pain) [109].

Oesophageal abnormalities included dysmotility and hypersensitivity. Oesophageal manometry and provocative testing are used to diagnose NCCP due to oesophageal motility disorder. Several tests, such as balloon distension, acid perfusion test, impedance planimetry and electrical stimulation can be used to determine the presence of oesophageal hypersensitivity in NCCP patients, although most are not used routinely in clinical practice [110]. But, well-known symptoms in pulmonary disorders are dyspnoea, cough and wheezing, whereas other symptoms such as fatigue, nausea and insomnia [111]. Finally, psychological factors are discussed if the diagnosis is not based on any of organic factors. In general, it seems that the use of a flag system could facilitate the diagnostic process allowing systematic assessment of first red flags (acute disease requiring immediate diagnosis and care), then green flags (identifiable diseases), and yellow flags (psychological diseases) [3].

Differentiated Impact of Pain with Organic or Psychological Origin

Chest pain resulting from physical origin can be cured in case of identifying the origin of the pain. Thus, the patient concerns about the cause of chest pain will be reduced. But, the patient becomes confused if a physical cause cannot be found. Although in these cases are raised psychological causes, it is extremely difficult to convince patients. Factors such as depression, anxiety, and stress are effective not only in the genesis of chest pain, but are leading to intensified pain [108]. According to a recent report, the cause of pain in 41 percent of patients is related to psychological factors [108] that unfortunately in 83% of cases are not diagnosed [82]. This leads to continued concern, repeated visits to the emergency department, and the imposition of additional costs to the patient and healthcare system [100].

NCCP Outcomes and Psychological Distress

Patients with NCCP are forced into a hard life involuntarily and this issue affects their social activities and interpersonal relationship; in addition to causing stress, anxiety and fear [112], which interfere in their physical performance [113] and quality of life [114]. According to some reports [115, 116], it has been known that despite positive prognosis on the mortality and the risk of cardiac complication development in these patients, in 1-11-year follow up post-cardiac examinations, more than 70 percent of them still have regular pain and in 50 percent of them, a belief exists that this pain is in fact a cardiac problem. Of this, 71 to 79 percent are regularly examined by a cardiologist and receive care and medication. The cross-sectional studies on patients with NCCP have shown the relationship between this issue and psychological distress, high rate of concomitant psychiatric disorders, suicidal thoughts, job impotency, disordered functions and quality of life alonwith irregular taking of medicinal drugs [96, 117]. According to Zincir *et al.* (2014), in comparison with angina pectoris, there is a relationship between NCCP and disorder in daily performance (including work, walking, exercise, and housekeeping activities), lowered quality of life and increase in occupational and social disabilities [118]. Furthermore, these patients experience high rates of stress and depression, take more leave days at their job and their social life is intensively under the impact of this pain [86]. The intensity of weakness and disability in this group of patient is in such a degree that according to the reports, nearly 50 percent of them are unable to perform their personal work and express disabilities extensively due to the pain [107].

Despite the absence of cardiac or physical etiologies for pain in NCCP patients and desirable cardiac prognosis [9], both pain and related problems such as stress, anxiety, avoidance behavior and the necessity to receive frequent assurance remain in most patients for long time. These conditions might be due to occupational and performance disabilities and frequent use of health services [119], and/or the consequences of poor perception of patients on the nature of their illness. These patients usually have poor perception of their current status and those conditions usually facilitate the development of psychological consequences. According to the reports of Zincir *et al.* (2014), patients whose pains have non-cardiac origin, in comparison with patients experiencing cardiac-related pain, believe their situation to be less understandable and less controllable; and they mostly experience higher health-related stress [118]. The illness perception in these patients has a negative relationship with their depression, stress, intensity of chest pain and interference in their daily life [120], as much as each one of these psychological factors including perceptional, emotional and behavioral factors is able to affect their perception of pain. Hence, the pathological process of the individual's complaints significantly affects the process of illness [121].

Dysfunctional thoughts and irrational beliefs serve as one of the psychological factors that affect the person's perception. Most NCCP patients have developed an inaccurate belief that the pain would lead to heart attack. In addition, pain causes fear of existence of a serious disease and even death. Hence, due to the emergence of an inaccurate diagnosis for pain patients keep interpreting their pain in a bad way [112]. In this line, studies of Bahremand *et al.* (2015) showed that patients with severe NCCP, in comparison with patients with mild pain, show more irrational beliefs and suffer more from emotional irresponsibility, distress in changes and avoidance from facing problems [94].

Other findings show that although NCCP patients use problem-centered approaches in solving their conflicts, their contrastive styles compared to healthy people are hard and inflexible [97]. This problem causes NCCP patients to experience higher degrees of stress, lower quality of life, higher periods of chest pain and more frequent use of medical and health services in long term despite having a healthy heart [122]. According to Webster *et al.* (2014), there is a relationship between perceived psychological factors and the psychological distress and sustained NCCP could lead to the development of depression, stress and low mental quality of life [123].

In spite of high rate of psychological symptoms in these patients and the relationship between higher rates of depression and anxiety with more use of health care services by these patients [86, 114], around 75 percent of specialists do not show serious attention to the psychological disorders in patients such as depression, stress, obsession, and physical complaints [124]. This absence of will to study psychological problems causes more frequent visits of those patients to the medical offices and clinics which might lead to crowds of patients and lack of proper screening of actual cardiac patients. On the other hand, it has been shown that physician's assurance provided for the patients with the goal of reducing patient's stress and frequent visits [125] does not yield patient's confidence and peace [126]. Therefore, more interventions are required for providing support and completing the initial assurance.

NCCP and Psychotherapy

The NCCP pathophysiology is highly complicated and seldom understandable. Therefore, the treatment of this problem is hard and challenging due to its heterogeneous nature. A usual approach is to teach patients and make them aware of "the nature of development" of NCCP and positive prognosis on the mortality caused by it in comparison with CCP [119, 127]. Furthermore, it is recommended to arrange the treatment to aim at lowering unnecessary use of medical emergency services and other medical resources than reducing the emergence and intensity of chest pain symptoms as well as improving the quality of life of patients [100]. Nevertheless, psychotherapy could follow its specific goals. The goal of psychotherapy is initially improving the patients' beliefs and cognitions, followed by developing adaptability behaviors [94]. Psychotherapy and in particular cognitive-behavioral therapies (CBTs) for this group of patients aims at correcting their dysfunctional perspectives on pathogenesis and risky nature of their physical symptoms (that is, chest pain). Patients must admit that psychological factors are the causes of their developing pains with non-physical origin and attribute that pain to panic attacks, stress and other psychological factors. The three general principles which are adopted in cognitive-behavioral treatment process are: 1) to provide a non-cardiac explanations for the symptoms that the patients manifest through showing the problems as a composition of physical, cognitive and behavioral factors and challenging any tragic interpretation of symptoms in patients; 2) to teach patients on the ways to overcome their symptoms by using behavioral interventions such as relaxation and breathing control; and 3) to show potential problems emerging from everlasting problems such as stress, family, work or other personal problems [100].

Controlled clinical trials on treating NCCP have shown that these relatively extensive interventions have been effective in reducing psychological distress, periods of chest pain frequency and lowering functional problems. Psychotherapy; especially cognitive- behavioral interventions [128] are generally designed by aiming at managing and controlling irrational beliefs and stress [82]. These interventions can have significant effects in lowering the pain [128 - 133] and psychological distress [128, 129, 134, 135]. Due to changes in dysfunctional perspectives and irrational beliefs, cognitive treatments help these patients [94] and perhaps change patients' views on pain. In this approach, Klimes *et al.* (1990) studied the effectiveness of cognitive therapy (CT) on reducing symptoms of NCCP patients. The results of the study showed that CT is significantly effective in lowering chest pain, confusions in daily life, autonomic symptoms and distress associated with psychological comorbidities and the improvement remains effective in the subsequent six-month follow-up [136]. Mayou *et al.* (1997) in their psychological studies on this group of patients showed that this treatment has been effective in reducing limitations in activities, concerns on physical symptoms and improving mood [137]. In this line, the results of another study showed that CT is effective in reducing fear caused by physical sensations, acceptable rate of thought in connection with the illness, negative self-developing thoughts and trends to take a tragic interpretation of physical feelings in NCCP patients [138].

According to Potts *et al.* (1999), CT is significantly effective in reducing chest pain, stress and depression in NCCP patients and the improvement sustains in the subsequent six months as well [139]. Ultimately, two more studies showed that CT, whether in group therapy or individually, is effective in reducing the symptoms of NCCP patients [130, 140].

Behavior therapies, which are mostly employed along with cognitive interventions, cover an extensive spectrum of methods. Relaxation training is one of those methods that in addition to reducing the intensity of pain in patients, is able to correct their irrational beliefs as well [82]. Relaxation training in NCCP patients could significantly reduce their depression, stress and frequency of their chest pain and its effects sustain for the next six months as well [139]. Diaphragmatic breathing, hypnotherapy and bio-feedback are also among prevalent interventions. The results of a study on diaphragmatic breathing effects on this group of patients showed that this treatment was effective in improving breathing rate and carbon dioxide levels and reducing the pain rate in a three-year follow up [141]. In addition, the results of a study showed the effectiveness of bio-feedback in reducing the symptoms of NCCP patients [142]. Teaching coping skills and cognitive contrastive approaches are among other methods that are able to significantly reduce stress, physical symptoms and complaints of pain, tragic view of pain and intensity of the pain [143, 144].

CONFLICT OF INTEREST

The authors confirm that they have no conflict of interest to declare for this publication.

ACKNOWLEDGEMENTS

Declared none.

REFERENCES

[1] White KS. Assessment and treatment of psychological causes of chest pain. Med Clin North Am 2010; 94(2): 291-318.

[http://dx.doi.org/10.1016/j.mcna.2010.01.005] [PMID: 20380957]

[2] Fass R, Achem SR. Noncardiac chest pain: epidemiology, natural course and pathogenesis. J Neurogastroenterol Motil 2011; 17(2): 110-23.
[http://dx.doi.org/10.5056/jnm.2011.17.2.110] [PMID: 21602987]

[3] Wertli MM, Ruchti KB, Steurer J, Held U. Diagnostic indicators of non-cardiovascular chest pain: a systematic review and meta-analysis. BMC Med 2013; 11: 239.
[http://dx.doi.org/10.1186/1741-7015-11-239] [PMID: 24207111]

[4] Eslick GD, Jones MP, Talley NJ. Non-cardiac chest pain: prevalence, risk factors, impact and consulting--a population-based study. Aliment Pharmacol Ther 2003; 17(9): 1115-24.
[http://dx.doi.org/10.1046/j.1365-2036.2003.01557.x] [PMID: 12752348]

[5] Cheung TK, Hou X, Lam KF, *et al.* Quality of life and psychological impact in patients with noncardiac chest pain. J Clin Gastroenterol 2009; 43(1): 13-8.
[http://dx.doi.org/10.1097/MCG.0b013e3181514725] [PMID: 18698264]

[6] Jonsbu E, Dammen T, Morken G, Martinsen EW. Patients with noncardiac chest pain and benign palpitations referred for cardiac outpatient investigation: a 6-month follow-up. Gen Hosp Psychiatry 2010; 32(4): 406-12.
[http://dx.doi.org/10.1016/j.genhosppsych.2010.03.003] [PMID: 20633745]

[7] Jerlock M, Kjellgren KI, Gaston-Johansson F, *et al.* Psychosocial profile in men and women with unexplained chest pain. J Intern Med 2008; 264(3): 265-74.
[http://dx.doi.org/10.1111/j.1365-2796.2008.01961.x] [PMID: 18397246]

[8] Kahn SE. The challenge of evaluating the patient with chest pain. Arch Pathol Lab Med 2000; 124(10): 1418-9.
[PMID: 11035567]

[9] Schroeder S, Schmid S, Martin A. Illness representations in non-cardiac chest pain – a Brief Behavioral Medical Intervention. Verhaltenstherapie 2013; 23: 234-42.

[10] Gaziano TA, Gaziano JM. Global Burden of Cardiovascular Disease. In: Bonow RO, Mann DL, Zipes DP, Libby P, Braunwald E, Eds. Braunwald's Heart disease: A text book of cardiovascular medicine. 9th ed., Philadelphia: Saunders 2012.
[http://dx.doi.org/10.1016/B978-1-4377-0398-6.00001-9]

[11] Sheps DS, Creed F, Clouse RE. Chest pain in patients with cardiac and noncardiac disease. Psychosom Med 2004; 66(6): 861-7.
[http://dx.doi.org/10.1097/01.psy.0000146330.80895.77] [PMID: 15564350]

[12] Sabatine MS, Cannon CP. Approach to the Patient with Chest Pain. In: Bonow RO, Mann DL, Zipes DP, Libby P, Braunwald E, Eds. Braunwald's Heart disease: A text book of cardiovascular medicine. 9th ed. Philadelphia: Saunders 2012; pp. 1076-7.
[http://dx.doi.org/10.1016/B978-1-4377-0398-6.00053-6]

[13] Nasiłowska-Barud A, Fedorovich V, Zapolski T, Sikorska-Jaroszyńska M, Wysokiński A. Pain-coping strategies in women with ischemic heart disease. Ann Agric Environ Med 2013; 20(4): 767-72.
[PMID: 24364450]

[14] Erdling A, Bondesson S, Pettersson T, Edvinsson L. Enhanced external counter pulsation in treatment

of refractory angina pectoris: two year outcome and baseline factors associated with treatment failure. BMC Cardiovasc Disord 2008; 8: 39.
[http://dx.doi.org/10.1186/1471-2261-8-39] [PMID: 19094202]

[15] Modi M, Ishimori ML, Sandhu VK, Wallace DJ, Weisman MH. Chest pain in lupus patients: the emergency department experience. Clin Rheumatol 2015; 34(11): 1969-73.
[http://dx.doi.org/10.1007/s10067-015-2948-4] [PMID: 25912215]

[16] Ruigómez A, Rodríguez LA, Wallander MA, Johansson S, Jones R. Chest pain in general practice: incidence, comorbidity and mortality. Fam Pract 2006; 23(2): 167-74.
[http://dx.doi.org/10.1093/fampra/cmi124] [PMID: 16461444]

[17] Casey DP, Beck DT, Nichols WW, *et al.* Effects of enhanced external counterpulsation on arterial stiffness and myocardial oxygen demand in patients with chronic angina pectoris. Am J Cardiol 2011; 107(10): 1466-72.
[http://dx.doi.org/10.1016/j.amjcard.2011.01.021] [PMID: 21420062]

[18] Parikh R, Kadowitz PJ. Angina pectoris: current therapy and future treatment options. Expert Rev Cardiovasc Ther 2014; 12(2): 175-86.
[http://dx.doi.org/10.1586/14779072.2014.880339] [PMID: 24417454]

[19] Tousoulis D, Androulakis E, Kontogeorgou A, *et al.* Insight to the pathophysiology of stable angina pectoris. Curr Pharm Des 2013; 19(9): 1593-600.
[PMID: 23016715]

[20] Ketterer MW, Bekkouche NS, Goldberg AD, McMahon RP, Krantz DS. Symptoms of anxiety and depression are correlates of angina pectoris by recent history and an ischemia-positive treadmill test in patients with documented coronary artery disease in the pimi study 2011.
[http://dx.doi.org/10.1155/2011/134040]

[21] Schiffer F, Hartley LH, Schulman CL, Abelmann WH. Evidence for emotionally-induced coronary arterial spasm in patients with angina pectoris. Br Heart J 1980; 44(1): 62-6.
[http://dx.doi.org/10.1136/hrt.44.1.62] [PMID: 7426162]

[22] Foreman RD, Garrett KM, Blair RW. Mechanisms of cardiac pain. Compr Physiol 2015; 5(2): 929-60.
[http://dx.doi.org/10.1002/cphy.c140032] [PMID: 25880519]

[23] Marzilli M, Merz CN, Boden WE, *et al.* Obstructive coronary atherosclerosis and ischemic heart disease: an elusive link! J Am Coll Cardiol 2012; 60(11): 951-6.
[http://dx.doi.org/10.1016/j.jacc.2012.02.082] [PMID: 22954239]

[24] Kothawade K, Bairey Merz CN. Microvascular coronary dysfunction in women: pathophysiology, diagnosis, and management. Curr Probl Cardiol 2011; 36(8): 291-318.
[http://dx.doi.org/10.1016/j.cpcardiol.2011.05.002] [PMID: 21723447]

[25] Hofkamp SE, Henrikson CA, Wegener ST. An interactive model of pain and myocardial ischemia. Psychosom Med 2007; 69(7): 632-9.
[http://dx.doi.org/10.1097/PSY.0b013e318151a4bd] [PMID: 17766689]

[26] Freedland KE, Carney RM, Krone RJ, Case NB, Case RB. Psychological determinants of anginal pain perception during exercise testing of stable patients after recovery from acute myocardial infarction or unstable angina pectoris. Am J Cardiol 1996; 77(1): 1-4.

[http://dx.doi.org/10.1016/S0002-9149(97)89124-2] [PMID: 8540443]

[27] Furze G, Lewin RJ, Murberg T, Bull P, Thompson DR. Does it matter what patients think? The relationship between changes in patients' beliefs about angina and their psychological and functional status. J Psychosom Res 2005; 59(5): 323-9.
[http://dx.doi.org/10.1016/j.jpsychores.2005.06.071] [PMID: 16253623]

[28] Strike PC, Steptoe A. Systematic review of mental stress-induced myocardial ischaemia. Eur Heart J 2003; 24(8): 690-703.
[http://dx.doi.org/10.1016/S0195-668X(02)00615-2] [PMID: 12713764]

[29] Vaccarino V, Bremner JD. Psychiatric and Behavioral Aspects of Cardiovascular Disease. In: Bonow RO, Mann DL, Zipes DP, Libby P, Braunwald E. editors. Braunwald's Heart disease: A text book of cardiovascular medicine. 9nd ed. Philadelphia Saunders 2012. pp. 1908.

[30] Hecht HS, DeBord L, Sotomayor N, Shaw R, Ryan C. Truly silent ischemia and the relationship of chest pain and ST segment changes to the amount of ischemic myocardium: evaluation by supine bicycle stress echocardiography. J Am Coll Cardiol 1994; 23(2): 369-76.
[http://dx.doi.org/10.1016/0735-1097(94)90422-7] [PMID: 8294689]

[31] Braverman AC, Thompson RW, Sanchez LA. Diseases of the Aorta. In: Bonow RO, Mann DL, Zipes DP, Libby P, Braunwald E, Eds. Braunwald's Heart disease: A text book of cardiovascular medicine. 9th ed. Philadelphia: Saunders 2012; pp. 1310-9.
[http://dx.doi.org/10.1016/B978-1-4377-0398-6.00060-3]

[32] Golledge J, Hankey GJ, Yeap BB, Almeida OP, Flicker L, Norman PE. Reported high salt intake is associated with increased prevalence of abdominal aortic aneurysm and larger aortic diameter in older men. PLoS One 2014; 9(7): e102578.
[http://dx.doi.org/10.1371/journal.pone.0102578] [PMID: 25036037]

[33] von Dohlen TW, Rogers WB, Frank MJ. Pathophysiology and management of unstable angina. Clin Cardiol 1989; 12(7): 363-9.
[http://dx.doi.org/10.1002/clc.4960120703] [PMID: 2568205]

[34] Silva LM, Barbirato GB, Drumond Neto C, Nobrega AC, Coimbra A, Mesquita CT. Reported high salt intake is associated with increased prevalence of abdominal aortic aneurysm and larger aortic diameter in older men. PLoS One Radionuclide imaging of myocardium with mental stress in the investigation of thoracic pain 2014; 9: e1025-78.

[35] Lewin B. The psychological and behavioral management of angina. J Psychosom Res 1997; 43(5): 453-62.
[http://dx.doi.org/10.1016/S0022-3999(97)00143-8] [PMID: 9394261]

[36] Blumenthal JA, Jiang W, Babyak MA, *et al.* Stress management and exercise training in cardiac patients with myocardial ischemia. Effects on prognosis and evaluation of mechanisms. Arch Intern Med 1997; 157(19): 2213-23.
[http://dx.doi.org/10.1001/archinte.1997.00440400063008] [PMID: 9342998]

[37] Lenfant C. Chest pain of cardiac and noncardiac origin. Metabolism 2010; 59 (Suppl. 1): S41-6.
[http://dx.doi.org/10.1016/j.metabol.2010.07.014] [PMID: 20837193]

[38] Bekkouche NS, Wawrzyniak AJ, Whittaker KS, Ketterer MW, Krantz DS. Psychological and

physiological predictors of angina during exercise-induced ischemia in patients with coronary artery disease. Psychosom Med 2013; 75(4): 413-21.
[http://dx.doi.org/10.1097/PSY.0b013e31828c4cb4] [PMID: 23576766]

[39] Chen H, Zhang L, Zhang M, *et al.* Relationship of depression, stress and endothelial function in stable angina patients. Physiol Behav 2013; 118: 152-8.
[http://dx.doi.org/10.1016/j.physbeh.2013.05.024] [PMID: 23688945]

[40] Verthein U, Köhler T. The correlation between everyday stress and angina pectoris: a longitudinal study. J Psychosom Res 1997; 43(3): 241-5.
[http://dx.doi.org/10.1016/S0022-3999(97)00054-8] [PMID: 9304550]

[41] Pimple P, Shah AJ, Rooks C, *et al.* Angina and mental stress-induced myocardial ischemia. J Psychosom Res 2015; 78(5): 433-7.
[http://dx.doi.org/10.1016/j.jpsychores.2015.02.007] [PMID: 25727240]

[42] Sullivan MD, Ciechanowski PS, Russo JE, *et al.* Angina pectoris during daily activities and exercise stress testing: The role of inducible myocardial ischemia and psychological distress. Pain 2008; 139(3): 551-61.
[http://dx.doi.org/10.1016/j.pain.2008.06.009] [PMID: 18694624]

[43] Maddox TM, Reid KJ, Spertus JA, *et al.* Angina at 1 year after myocardial infarction: prevalence and associated findings. Arch Intern Med 2008; 168(12): 1310-6.
[http://dx.doi.org/10.1001/archinte.168.12.1310] [PMID: 18574088]

[44] Garganeeva NP, Petrova MM, Evsyukov AA, Shtarik SY, Kaskaeva DS. [The influence of depression on the course of coronary heart disease and quality of life]. Klin Med (Mosk) 2014; 92(12): 30-7.
[PMID: 25980296]

[45] Eken C, Oktay C, Bacanli A, *et al.* Anxiety and depressive disorders in patients presenting with chest pain to the emergency department: a comparison between cardiac and non-cardiac origin. J Emerg Med 2010; 39(2): 144-50.
[http://dx.doi.org/10.1016/j.jemermed.2007.11.087] [PMID: 18722737]

[46] Tsouna-Hadjis E, Kallergis G, Agrios N, *et al.* Pain intensity in nondiabetic patients with myocardial infarction or unstable angina. Its association with clinical and psychological features. Int J Cardiol 1998; 67(2): 165-9.
[http://dx.doi.org/10.1016/S0167-5273(98)00319-2] [PMID: 9891951]

[47] Lumley MA, Torosian T, Ketterer MW, Pickard SD. Psychosocial factors related to non-cardiac chest pain during treadmill exercise. Psychosomatics 1997; 38: S121-6.
[http://dx.doi.org/10.1016/S0033-3182(97)71459-2]

[48] Greenwood KA, Thurston R, Rumble M, Waters SJ, Keefe FJ. Anger and persistent pain: current status and future directions. Pain 2003; 103(1-2): 1-5.
[http://dx.doi.org/10.1016/S0304-3959(03)00132-5] [PMID: 12749952]

[49] Saeidi M. The efficacy methods of relaxation and reconstruction of cognitive on anxiety and depression in cardiac rehabilitation patients. Thesis of MA in psychology. Tehran Psychiatry Institute 2004.

[50] Komasi S. The effectiveness of tow methods of relaxation and interpersonal cognitive problem solving

(ICPS) on decreasing anxiety and depression in cardiac rehabilitation patients. Tonekabon: Islamic Azad university 2010.

[51] Soroush A, Heydarpour B, Saeidi M, Komasi S, Ezzati P, Rashidi AA. Cardiac Disease Risk Factors In Cardiac Rehabilitation Patients with and without Depression. 1st international congress of cardiac rehabilitation. Isfahan Iran1.

[52] Saeidi M, Komasi S, Soroush A, Zakiei A, Shakeri J. Gender Differences in Patients' Beliefs About Biological, Environmental, Behavioral, and Psychological Risk Factors in a Cardiac Rehabilitation Program. J Cardio-Thoracic Med 2014; 2: 215-20.

[53] Saeidi M, Soroush A, Komasi S, Momeni K, Heydarpour B. Attitudes Toward Cardiovascular Disease Risk Factors Among Patients Referred to a Cardiac Rehabilitation Center: Importance of Psychological Attitudes. Shiraz E Med J 2015; 16(7): e22281.

[54] Perkins-Porras L, Whitehead DL, Steptoe A. Patients' beliefs about the causes of heart disease: relationships with risk factors, sex and socio-economic status. Eur J Cardiovasc Prev Rehabil 2006; 13(5): 724-30.
[http://dx.doi.org/10.1097/01.hjr.0000216551.81882.11] [PMID: 17001211]

[55] McCabe PJ, Barnason SA, Houfek J. Illness beliefs in patients with recurrent symptomatic atrial fibrillation. Pacing Clin Electrophysiol 2011; 34(7): 810-20.
[http://dx.doi.org/10.1111/j.1540-8159.2011.03105.x] [PMID: 21507022]

[56] van der Wal MH, Jaarsma T, Moser DK, Veeger NJ, van Gilst WH, van Veldhuisen DJ. Compliance in heart failure patients: the importance of knowledge and beliefs. Eur Heart J 2006; 27(4): 434-40.
[http://dx.doi.org/10.1093/eurheartj/ehi603] [PMID: 16230302]

[57] Channer KS, O'Connor S, Britton S, Walbridge D, Rees JR. Psychological factors influence the success of coronary artery surgery. J R Soc Med 1988; 81(11): 629-32.
[PMID: 3264855]

[58] Sobanski JA, Klasa K, Popiolek L, *et al.* Complaints of patients suffering from neurotic disorders, interesting for cardiologist. Kardiol Pol 2015.

[59] Ronaldson A, Poole L, Kidd T, Leigh E, Jahangiri M, Steptoe A. Optimism measured pre-operatively is associated with reduced pain intensity and physical symptom reporting after coronary artery bypass graft surgery. J Psychosom Res 2014; 77(4): 278-82.
[http://dx.doi.org/10.1016/j.jpsychores.2014.07.018] [PMID: 25129850]

[60] Park MS, Lee KH, Sohn S, Eom JS, Sohn JH. Degree of extraversion and physiological responses to physical pain and sadness. Scand J Psychol 2014; 55(5): 483-8.
[http://dx.doi.org/10.1111/sjop.12144] [PMID: 25040459]

[61] Etherton J, Lawson M, Graham R. Individual and gender differences in subjective and objective indices of pain: gender, fear of pain, pain catastrophizing and cardiovascular reactivity. Appl Psychophysiol Biofeedback 2014; 39(2): 89-97.
[http://dx.doi.org/10.1007/s10484-014-9245-x] [PMID: 24696322]

[62] Schroeder S, Achenbach S, Körber S, Nowy K, de Zwaan M, Martin A. Cognitive-perceptual factors in noncardiac chest pain and cardiac chest pain. Psychosom Med 2012; 74(8): 861-8.
[http://dx.doi.org/10.1097/PSY.0b013e31826ae4ae] [PMID: 23006429]

[63] Kimble LP, Dunbar SB, Weintraub WS, McGuire DB, Manzo SF, Strickland OL. Symptom clusters and health-related quality of life in people with chronic stable angina. J Adv Nurs 2011; 67(5): 1000-11.
[http://dx.doi.org/10.1111/j.1365-2648.2010.05564.x] [PMID: 21352270]

[64] Muhlestein JB, Grehan S. Ranolazine reduces patient-reported angina severity and frequency and improves quality of life in selected patients with chronic angina. Drugs R D 2013; 13(3): 207-13.
[http://dx.doi.org/10.1007/s40268-013-0026-4] [PMID: 23990357]

[65] Safdar B, Foody JM, D'Onofrio G. Depression as modifiable coronary risk factor in the emergency department chest pain observation unit: a pilot. Crit Pathw Cardiol 2010; 9(2): 82-7.
[http://dx.doi.org/10.1097/HPC.0b013e3181db06ef] [PMID: 20520215]

[66] Serber ER, Edwards-Hampton SA, Yeager B, *et al.* Prevalence of Chest Pain, Depression, Somatization, Anxiety, Global Distress, and Substance Use among Cardiac and Pulmonary Rehabilitation Patients. Pain Res Treat 2012; 2012: 138680.

[67] Nezu AM, Nezu CM, Jain D, *et al.* Social problem solving and noncardiac chest pain. Psychosom Med 2007; 69(9): 944-51.
[http://dx.doi.org/10.1097/PSY.0b013e31815a995a] [PMID: 17991820]

[68] Thieme K, Turk DC, Gracely RH, Maixner W, Flor H. The relationship among psychological and psychophysiological characteristics of fibromyalgia patients. J Pain 2015; 16(2): 186-96.
[http://dx.doi.org/10.1016/j.jpain.2014.11.009] [PMID: 25433166]

[69] Zengin S, Kabul S, Al B, Sarcan E, Doğan M, Yildirim C. Effects of music therapy on pain and anxiety in patients undergoing port catheter placement procedure. Complement Ther Med 2013; 21(6): 689-96.
[http://dx.doi.org/10.1016/j.ctim.2013.08.017] [PMID: 24280479]

[70] Akyildiz ZI, Ergene O. Frequency of angina and quality of life in outpatients with stable coronary artery disease in Turkey: insights from the PULSE study. Acta Cardiol 2014; 69(3): 253-9.
[PMID: 25029869]

[71] Moattari M, Adib F, Kojuri J, Tabatabaee SH. Angina self-management plan and quality of life, anxiety and depression in post coronary angioplasty patients. Iran Red Crescent Med J 2014; 16(11): e16981.
[PMID: 25763214]

[72] McGillion M, Arthur H, Victor JC, Watt-Watson J, Cosman T. Effectiveness of Psychoeducational Interventions for Improving Symptoms, Health-Related Quality of Life, and Psychological well Being in Patients with Stable Angina. Curr Cardiol Rev 2008; 4(1): 1-11.
[http://dx.doi.org/10.2174/157340308783565393] [PMID: 19924272]

[73] Ballegaard S, Petersen PB, Harboe GS, Karpatschof B, Gyntelberg F, Faber J. The association between changes in pressure pain sensitivity and changes in cardiovascular physiological factors associated with persistent stress. Scand J Clin Lab Invest 2014; 74(2): 116-25.
[http://dx.doi.org/10.3109/00365513.2013.862847] [PMID: 24313546]

[74] Koenig J, Loerbroks A, Jarczok MN, Fischer JE, Thayer JF. Chronic Pain and Heart Rate Variability in a Cross-Sectional Occupational Sample: Evidence for Impaired Vagal Control. Clin J Pain 2015.

[http://dx.doi.org/10.1111/pme.12825] [PMID: 25924095]

[75] Hampton AJ, Hadjistavropoulos T, Gagnon MM, Williams J, Clark D. The effects of emotion regulation strategies on the pain experience: a structured laboratory investigation. Pain 2015; 156(5): 868-79.
[http://dx.doi.org/10.1097/j.pain.0000000000000126] [PMID: 25734999]

[76] Karami J, Komasi S, Maesoomi M, Saeidi M. Comparing the effects of two methods of relaxation and interpersonal cognitive problem solving (ICPS) on decreasing anxiety and depression in cardiac rehabilitation patients. Urmia Med J 2014; 25: 298-308.

[77] Mosso-Vázquez JL, Gao K, Wiederhold BK, Wiederhold MD. Virtual reality for pain management in cardiac surgery. Cyberpsychol Behav Soc Netw 2014; 17(6): 371-8.
[http://dx.doi.org/10.1089/cyber.2014.0198] [PMID: 24892200]

[78] Sun J, Buys N, Jayasinghe R. Effects of community-based meditative Tai Chi programme on improving quality of life, physical and mental health in chronic heart-failure participants. Aging Ment Health 2014; 18(3): 289-95.
[http://dx.doi.org/10.1080/13607863.2013.875120] [PMID: 24404785]

[79] Zamunér AR, Andrade CP, Forti M, *et al.* Effects of a hydrotherapy programme on symbolic and complexity dynamics of heart rate variability and aerobic capacity in fibromyalgia patients. Clin Exp Rheumatol 2015; 33(1) (Suppl. 88): S73-81.
[PMID: 25786047]

[80] Roberts MH, Klatzkin RR, Mechlin B. Social Support Attenuates Physiological Stress Responses and Experimental Pain Sensitivity to Cold Pressor Pain. Ann Behav Med 2015; 49(4): 557-69.
[http://dx.doi.org/10.1007/s12160-015-9686-3] [PMID: 25623896]

[81] Komasi S, Saeidi M. Screening For Depressive Symptoms at the Beginning of Outpatient Cardiac Rehabilitation by Assessed Perceived Risk Factors by Patients. Clin Med Rev Case Rep 2015; 2(8).

[82] Bahremand M, Moradi G, Saeidi M, Mohammadi S, Komasi S. Reducing Irrational Beliefs and Pain Severity in Patients Suffering from Non-Cardiac Chest Pain (NCCP): A Comparison of Relaxation Training and Metaphor Therapy. Korean J Pain 2015; 28(2): 88-95.
[http://dx.doi.org/10.3344/kjp.2015.28.2.88] [PMID: 25852829]

[83] Zimmermann K, Einsle F, Dannemann S, Pollack K, Köllner V, Nitschke-Bertaud M. [Psychological and physical well-being of cardiological outpatients with chest pain]. Psychother Psychosom Med Psychol 2010; 60(9-10): 368-78. [Psychological and physical well-being of cardiological outpatients with chest pain].
[http://dx.doi.org/10.1055/s-0029-1243227] [PMID: 20094968]

[84] Eslick GD, Coulshed DS, Talley NJ. Review article: the burden of illness of non-cardiac chest pain. Aliment Pharmacol Ther 2002; 16(7): 1217-23.
[http://dx.doi.org/10.1046/j.1365-2036.2002.01296.x] [PMID: 12144570]

[85] Bringager CB, Friis S, Arnesen H, Dammen T. Nine-year follow-up of panic disorder in chest pain patients: clinical course and predictors of outcome. Gen Hosp Psychiatry 2008; 30(2): 138-46.
[http://dx.doi.org/10.1016/j.genhosppsych.2007.12.009] [PMID: 18291295]

[86] Wong WM, Lam KF, Cheng C, *et al.* Population based study of noncardiac chest pain in southern

Chinese: prevalence, psychosocial factors and health care utilization. World J Gastroenterol 2004; 10(5): 707-12.
[http://dx.doi.org/10.3748/wjg.v10.i5.707] [PMID: 14991943]

[87] Chiocca JC, Olmos JA, Salis GB, Soifer LO, Higa R, Marcolongo M. Prevalence, clinical spectrum and atypical symptoms of gastro-oesophageal reflux in Argentina: a nationwide population-based study. Aliment Pharmacol Ther 2005; 22(4): 331-42.
[http://dx.doi.org/10.1111/j.1365-2036.2005.02565.x] [PMID: 16098000]

[88] Rey E, Elola-Olaso CM, Rodríguez-Artalejo F, Locke GR III, Díaz-Rubio M. Prevalence of atypical symptoms and their association with typical symptoms of gastroesophageal reflux in Spain. Eur J Gastroenterol Hepatol 2006; 18(9): 969-75.
[http://dx.doi.org/10.1097/01.meg.0000230081.53298.03] [PMID: 16894310]

[89] Eslick GD, Fass R. Noncardiac chest pain: evaluation and treatment. Gastroenterol Clin North Am 2003; 32(2): 531-52.
[http://dx.doi.org/10.1016/S0889-8553(03)00029-3] [PMID: 12858605]

[90] Jerlock M. Patients with unexplained chest pain: Pain experience, stress, coping and health-related quality of life. Sweden: Institute of Health and Care Sciences 2007.

[91] Glombiewski JA, Rief W, Bösner S, Keller H, Martin A, Donner-Banzhoff N. The course of nonspecific chest pain in primary care: symptom persistence and health care usage. Arch Intern Med 2010; 170(3): 251-5.
[http://dx.doi.org/10.1001/archinternmed.2009.474] [PMID: 20142569]

[92] White KS, Raffa SD, Jakle KR, *et al.* Morbidity of DSM-IV Axis I disorders in patients with noncardiac chest pain: Psychiatric morbidity linked with increased pain and health care utilization. J Consult Clin Psychol 2008; 76(3): 422-30.
[http://dx.doi.org/10.1037/0022-006X.76.3.422] [PMID: 18540735]

[93] Gillies M, Batty GD, Jhund PS. Prior psychiatric hospitalization: an underappreciated risk factor for premature mortality among individuals with chest pain. Eur Heart J 2012; 33(7): 804-6.
[PMID: 22586709]

[94] Bahremand M, Saeidi M, Komasi S. Non-coronary patients with severe chest pain show more irrational beliefs compared patients with mild pain. Korean J Fam Med 2015; 36(4): 180-5.
[http://dx.doi.org/10.4082/kjfm.2015.36.4.180] [PMID: 26217482]

[95] Olden KW. The psychological aspects of noncardiac chest pain. Gastroenterol Clin North Am 2004; 33(1): 61-7.
[http://dx.doi.org/10.1016/S0889-8553(03)00130-4] [PMID: 15062438]

[96] Dammen T, Arnesen H, Ekeberg O, Husebye T, Friis S. Panic disorder in chest pain patients referred for cardiological outpatient investigation. J Intern Med 1999; 245(5): 497-507.
[http://dx.doi.org/10.1046/j.1365-2796.1999.00447.x] [PMID: 10363751]

[97] Cheng C, Wong WM, Lai KC, *et al.* Psychosocial factors in patients with noncardiac chest pain. Psychosom Med 2003; 65(3): 443-9.
[http://dx.doi.org/10.1097/01.PSY.0000041623.24456.99] [PMID: 12764218]

[98] Kuijpers PM, Denollet J, Lousberg R, Wellens HJ, Crijns H, Honig A. Validity of the hospital anxiety

and depression scale for use with patients with noncardiac chest pain. Psychosomatics 2003; 44(4): 329-35.
[http://dx.doi.org/10.1176/appi.psy.44.4.329] [PMID: 12832599]

[99] Fagring AJ, Kjellgren KI, Rosengren A, Lissner L, Manhem K, Welin C. Depression, anxiety, stress, social interaction and health-related quality of life in men and women with unexplained chest pain. BMC Public Health 2008; 8: 165.
[http://dx.doi.org/10.1186/1471-2458-8-165] [PMID: 18489751]

[100] Achem SR. Noncardiac chest pain-treatment approaches. Gastroenterol Clin North Am 2008; 37(4): 859-878, ix.
[http://dx.doi.org/10.1016/j.gtc.2008.09.013] [PMID: 19028322]

[101] Smeijers L, van de Pas H, Nyklicek I, Notten PJ, Pedersen SS, Kop WJ. The independent association of anxiety with non-cardiac chest pain. Psychol Health 2014; 29(3): 253-63.
[http://dx.doi.org/10.1080/08870446.2013.843681] [PMID: 24160441]

[102] Webster RA. Psychological distress in non-cardiac chest pain patients: An application of the common sense model of illness representations. UK: University of Sheffield 2012.

[103] Webster R, Norman P, Goodacre S, Thompson A. The prevalence and correlates of psychological outcomes in patients with acute non-cardiac chest pain: a systematic review. Emerg Med J 2012; 29(4): 267-73.
[http://dx.doi.org/10.1136/emermed-2011-200526] [PMID: 22034535]

[104] White KS, McDonnell CJ, Gervino EV. Alexithymia and anxiety sensitivity in patients with non-cardiac chest pain. J Behav Ther Exp Psychiatry 2011; 42(4): 432-9.
[http://dx.doi.org/10.1016/j.jbtep.2011.04.001] [PMID: 21570932]

[105] Eslick GD, Koloski NA, Talley NJ. Sexual, physical, verbal/emotional abuse and unexplained chest pain. Child Abuse Negl 2011; 35(8): 601-5.
[http://dx.doi.org/10.1016/j.chiabu.2011.04.007] [PMID: 21862127]

[106] Kuijpers PM, Denollet J, Wellens HJ, Crijns HM, Honig A. Noncardiac chest pain in the emergency department: the role of cardiac history, anxiety or depression and Type D personality. Eur J Cardiovasc Prev Rehabil 2007; 14(2): 273-9.
[http://dx.doi.org/10.1097/HJR.0b013e32801da0fc] [PMID: 17446807]

[107] Jones MP, Venketesan T, Wulsin LR. Evaluation of Noncardiac Chest Pain: Toward a Positive Diagnosis. Hosp Physician 1999; 6(7): 41-53.

[108] Bahremand M, Saeidi M, Takallo F, Komasi S. Comparison of Depression, Anxiety, and Stress Between Mild and Severe Non-cardiac Chest Pain. Thrita 2016; 5: e32752.
[http://dx.doi.org/10.5812/thrita.32752]

[109] Winzenberg T, Jones G, Callisaya M. Musculoskeletal chest wall pain. Aust Fam Physician 2015; 44(8): 540-4.
[PMID: 26510139]

[110] Hershcovici T, Achem SR, Jha LK, Fass R. Systematic review: the treatment of noncardiac chest pain. Aliment Pharmacol Ther 2012; 35(1): 5-14.
[http://dx.doi.org/10.1111/j.1365-2036.2011.04904.x] [PMID: 22077344]

[111] van Dam van Isselt EF, Groenewegen-Sipkema KH, Spruit-van Eijk M, *et al.* Pain in patients with COPD: a systematic review and meta-analysis. BMJ Open 2014; 4(9): e005898. [http://dx.doi.org/10.1136/bmjopen-2014-005898] [PMID: 25260370]

[112] Jerlock M, Gaston-Johansson F, Danielson E. Living with unexplained chest pain. J Clin Nurs 2005; 14(8): 956-64. [http://dx.doi.org/10.1111/j.1365-2702.2005.01195.x] [PMID: 16102147]

[113] Shelby RA, Somers TJ, Keefe FJ, *et al.* Pain catastrophizing in patients with noncardiac chest pain: relationships with pain, anxiety, and disability. Psychosom Med 2009; 71(8): 861-8. [http://dx.doi.org/10.1097/PSY.0b013e3181b49584] [PMID: 19737857]

[114] Hadlandsmyth K, White KS, Krone RJ. Quality of life in patients with non-CAD chest pain: associations to fear of pain and psychiatric disorder severity. J Clin Psychol Med Settings 2013; 20(3): 284-93. [http://dx.doi.org/10.1007/s10880-012-9347-7] [PMID: 23338745]

[115] Ockene IS, Shay MJ, Alpert JS, Weiner BH, Dalen JE. Unexplained chest pain in patients with normal coronary arteriograms: a follow-up study of functional status. N Engl J Med 1980; 303(22): 1249-52. [http://dx.doi.org/10.1056/NEJM198011273032201] [PMID: 7421961]

[116] Lantinga LJ, Sprafkin RP, McCroskery JH, Baker MT, Warner RA, Hill NE. One-year psychosocial follow-up of patients with chest pain and angiographically normal coronary arteries. Am J Cardiol 1988; 62(4): 209-13. [http://dx.doi.org/10.1016/0002-9149(88)90213-5] [PMID: 3400599]

[117] Fleet RP, Dupuis G, Marchand A, Burelle D, Arsenault A, Beitman BD. Panic disorder in emergency department chest pain patients: prevalence, comorbidity, suicidal ideation, and physician recognition. Am J Med 1996; 101(4): 371-80. [http://dx.doi.org/10.1016/S0002-9343(96)00224-0] [PMID: 8873507]

[118] Zincir SB, Sunbul M, Sunbul EA, *et al.* Evaluation of alexithymia, somatosensory sensitivity, and health anxiety levels in patients with noncardiac chest pain. Biomed Res Int 2014; 2014: 896183.

[119] Kim JH, Rhee PL. Recent advances in noncardiac chest pain in Korea. Gut Liver 2012; 6(1): 1-9. [http://dx.doi.org/10.5009/gnl.2012.6.1.1] [PMID: 22375165]

[120] Israel JI, White KS, Gervino EV. Illness perceptions, negative emotions, and pain in patients with noncardiac chest pain. J Clin Psychol Med Settings 2015; 22(1): 77-89. [http://dx.doi.org/10.1007/s10880-015-9419-6] [PMID: 25609578]

[121] Bass C, Mayou R. Chest pain. BMJ 2002; 325(7364): 588-91. [http://dx.doi.org/10.1136/bmj.325.7364.588] [PMID: 12228139]

[122] Eslick GD, Talley NJ. Natural history and predictors of outcome for non-cardiac chest pain: a prospective 4-year cohort study. Neurogastroenterol Motil 2008; 20(9): 989-97. [http://dx.doi.org/10.1111/j.1365-2982.2008.01133.x] [PMID: 18466221]

[123] Webster R, Norman P, Goodacre S, Thompson AR, McEachan RR. Illness representations, psychological distress and non-cardiac chest pain in patients attending an emergency department. Psychol Health 2014; 29(11): 1265-82. [http://dx.doi.org/10.1080/08870446.2014.923885] [PMID: 24831735]

[124] Castillo-Richmond A, Schneider RH, Alexander CN, *et al.* Effects of stress reduction on carotid atherosclerosis in hypertensive African Americans. Stroke 2000; 31(3): 568-73. [http://dx.doi.org/10.1161/01.STR.31.3.568] [PMID: 10700487]

[125] Donkin L, Ellis CJ, Powell R, Broadbent E, Gamble G, Petrie KJ. Illness perceptions predict reassurance following a negative exercise stress testing result. Psychol Health 2006; 21: 421-30. [http://dx.doi.org/10.1080/14768320500329292]

[126] McDonald IG, Daly J, Jelinek VM, Panetta F, Gutman JM. Opening Pandora's box: the unpredictability of reassurance by a normal test result. BMJ 1996; 313(7053): 329-32. [http://dx.doi.org/10.1136/bmj.313.7053.329] [PMID: 8760739]

[127] Beitman BD, Kushner MG, Basha I, Lamberti J, Mukerji V, Bartels K. Follow-up status of patients with angiographically normal coronary arteries and panic disorder. JAMA 1991; 265(12): 1545-9. [http://dx.doi.org/10.1001/jama.1991.03460120059036] [PMID: 1825675]

[128] Spinhoven P, Van der Does AJ, Van Dijk E, Van Rood YR. Heart-focused anxiety as a mediating variable in the treatment of noncardiac chest pain by cognitive-behavioral therapy and paroxetine. J Psychosom Res 2010; 69(3): 227-35. [http://dx.doi.org/10.1016/j.jpsychores.2010.02.005] [PMID: 20708444]

[129] Asbury EA, Kanji N, Ernst E, Barbir M, Collins P. Autogenic training to manage symptomology in women with chest pain and normal coronary arteries. Menopause 2009; 16(1): 60-5. [http://dx.doi.org/10.1097/gme.0b013e318184762e] [PMID: 18978640]

[130] Esler JL, Bock BC. Psychological treatments for noncardiac chest pain: recommendations for a new approach. J Psychosom Res 2004; 56(3): 263-9. [http://dx.doi.org/10.1016/S0022-3999(03)00515-4] [PMID: 15046961]

[131] Jones H, Cooper P, Miller V, Brooks N, Whorwell PJ. Treatment of non-cardiac chest pain: a controlled trial of hypnotherapy. Gut 2006; 55(10): 1403-8. [http://dx.doi.org/10.1136/gut.2005.086694] [PMID: 16627548]

[132] Kisely S, Campbell LA, Skerritt P. Psychological interventions for symptomatic management of non-specific chest pain in patients with normal coronary anatomy. Cochrane Database Syst Rev 2005; (1): CD004101. [PMID: 15674930]

[133] Tyni-Lenne R, Stryjan S, Eriksson B, Berglund M, Sylven C. Beneficial therapeutic effects of physical training and relaxation therapy in women with coronary syndrome X. Physiother Res Int 2002; 7(1): 35-43. [http://dx.doi.org/10.1002/pri.239] [PMID: 11992983]

[134] Asbury EA, Slattery C, Grant A, Evans L, Barbir M, Collins P. Cardiac rehabilitation for the treatment of women with chest pain and normal coronary arteries. Menopause 2008; 15(3): 454-60. [http://dx.doi.org/10.1097/gme.0b013e31815982eb] [PMID: 18188136]

[135] Jonsbu E, Dammen T, Morken G, Moum T, Martinsen EW. Short-term cognitive behavioral therapy for non-cardiac chest pain and benign palpitations: a randomized controlled trial. J Psychosom Res 2011; 70(2): 117-23. [http://dx.doi.org/10.1016/j.jpsychores.2010.09.013] [PMID: 21262413]

[136] Klimes I, Mayou RA, Pearce MJ, Coles L, Fagg JR. Psychological treatment for atypical non-cardiac chest pain: a controlled evaluation. Psychol Med 1990; 20(3): 605-11. [http://dx.doi.org/10.1017/S0033291700017116] [PMID: 2236369]

[137] Mayou RA, Bryant BM, Sanders D, Bass C, Klimes I, Forfar C. A controlled trial of cognitive behavioural therapy for non-cardiac chest pain. Psychol Med 1997; 27(5): 1021-31. [http://dx.doi.org/10.1017/S0033291797005254] [PMID: 9300508]

[138] van Peski-Oosterbaan AS, Spinhoven P, van der Does AJ, Bruschke AV. Noncardiac chest pain: interest in a medical psychological treatment. J Psychosom Res 1998; 45(5): 471-6. [http://dx.doi.org/10.1016/S0022-3999(97)00306-1] [PMID: 9835242]

[139] Potts SG, Lewin R, Fox KA, Johnstone EC. Group psychological treatment for chest pain with normal coronary arteries. QJM 1999; 92(2): 81-6. [http://dx.doi.org/10.1093/qjmed/92.2.81] [PMID: 10209659]

[140] Cott A, McCully J, Goldberg WM, Tanser PH, Parkinson W. Interdisciplinary treatment of morbidity in benign chest pain. Angiology 1992; 43(3 Pt 1): 195-202. [http://dx.doi.org/10.1177/000331979204300304] [PMID: 1575367]

[141] DeGuire S, Gevirtz R, Hawkinson D, Dixon K. Breathing retraining: a three-year follow-up study of treatment for hyperventilation syndrome and associated functional cardiac symptoms. Biofeedback Self Regul 1996; 21(2): 191-8. [http://dx.doi.org/10.1007/BF02284695] [PMID: 8805966]

[142] Ryan M, Gevirtz R. Biofeedback-based psychophysiological treatment in a primary care setting: an initial feasibility study. Appl Psychophysiol Biofeedback 2004; 29(2): 79-93. [http://dx.doi.org/10.1023/B:APBI.0000026635.03016.ef] [PMID: 15208972]

[143] Keefe FJ, Shelby RA, Somers TJ, *et al.* Effects of coping skills training and sertraline in patients with non-cardiac chest pain: a randomized controlled study. Pain 2011; 152(4): 730-41. [http://dx.doi.org/10.1016/j.pain.2010.08.040] [PMID: 21324590]

[144] Lipsitz JD, Gur M, Albano AM, Sherman B. A psychological intervention for pediatric chest pain: development and open trial. J Dev Behav Pediatr 2011; 32(2): 153-7. [http://dx.doi.org/10.1097/DBP.0b013e318206d5aa] [PMID: 21200331]

CHAPTER 4

Genetic Explorations of Pain

Harjot Dhillon and **Puneetpal Singh***

Department of Human Genetics, Punjabi University, Patiala-147002, India

Abstract: Pain is the most prevalent form of human health malady which, if remain unaddressed, exerts formidable impact. Pain research has tried hard to unravel the possibilities in the direction of diagnosis and management of pain conditions, but knowledge of genetic consequences of pain is still in infancy. During pain, sensory input is realized, processed and regulated, first and foremost through ones genetic composition and then different characters of physiology, psychology, sociology and environment come in the scene. The present exposition demonstrates the precise details of various genes and genetic variants that participate in different phases of pain and pain conditions, disseminating an idea that in future, diagnosis and treatment of pain by harnessing indepth genetic knowledge has startling revelations in store for us.

Keywords: Chronic pain, Conduction, Genes, Modulation, Synaptic transmission, Transduction.

INTRODUCTION

Pain is a complex sensation where sensory, affective and cognitive dimensions of pain alongwith parallel neural networks in brain are associated with constellation of factors. Though pain occurs to show protective gesture, but when it surpasses threshold, exerts debilitating effect upon health and triggers concomitant physiological and psychological concerns of perilous ramifications. Right from the activation of primary afferent nociceptors upto the cortical processing of the pain in the higher regions of the brain, pain trajectory can be dissected into transduction, conduction, synaptic transmission and modulation.

* **Coresponding author Puneetpal Singh:** Department of Human Genetics, Punjabi University, Patiala; Email: singh.puneet@rediffmail.com

Besides, environmental, behavioral and psychological risks involved, all these stages of pain sensitivity, severity and analgesic responses are mediated by different sets of genes and genetic variants.

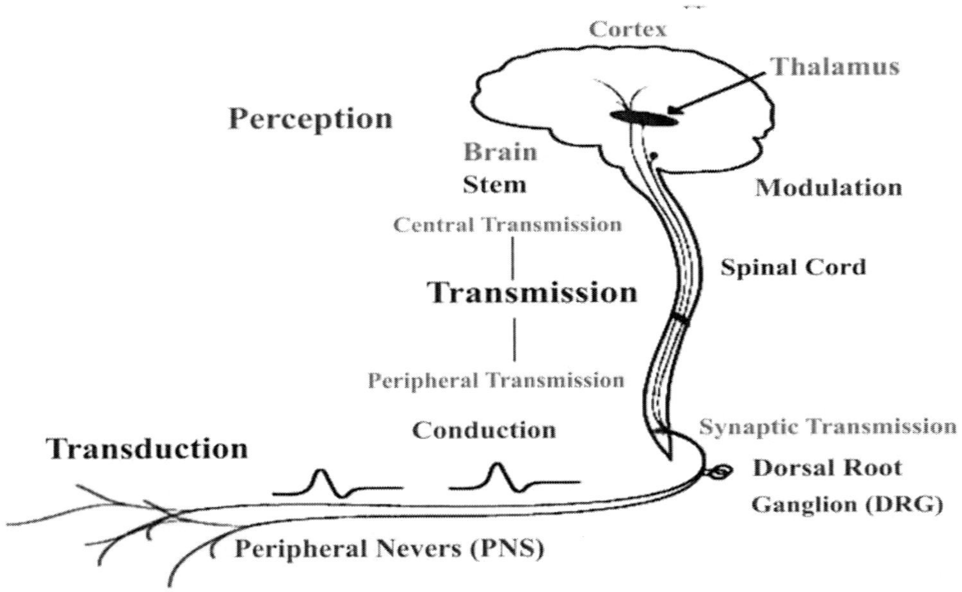

Fig. (1). Showing different phases of pain

1. TRANSDUCTION

Transduction marks the cardinal process for the pain realization. It involves detection of noxious stimuli by the peripheral nociceptors by sensing various substances such as substance P, bradykinin, *etc.* leading to the depolarization of the neurons causing generation of a receptor potential [1].

Heat Pain

The nociceptors detect four major types of noxious stimuli namely; heat, cold, mechanical and chemical. The detection of these various types of stimuli is further regulated by numerous genes. Amongst the most studied one in relation to heat related sensitization are the transient receptor potential (TRP) family genes. TRP family is a calcium gated channel protein family comprising 6 subfamilies; TRPA, TRPV, TRPM, TRPML, TRPP and TRPL. While the majority of TRP gene family members detect specific types of noxious insults, some of them are polymodal in function. A class of TRP gene family; TRPV1 is activated by both heat and capsaicin found in hot chilli pepper [2]. It is highly associated with detection of thermal, mechanical and pH shifts. The polymodal function of TRPV1 has been confirmed by various gene knockouts, siRNA knockout and inhibition studies [3]. In human, TRPV1 Met315Ile and Ile585Val polymorphism has been examined and Met315lle is found to be associated with greater susceptibility to chronic neuropathic pain [4]. TRPV1 acts in close amity with Protein kinase beta type II (PKCβII), as the activation of the latter by TRPV1 causes phosphorylation of Thr705, setting the pain and itch thresholds below normal ranges [5]. TRPV1 also regulates calcitonin gene related peptide (CGRP) functioning as TRPV1 knockouts show enhanced metabolism and longevity due to suppression of CGRP activity [6].The TRPV1 knockout shows reduced thermal sensitivity while TRPV2 knockout shows normal function. Surprisingly, 1911A>G (rs8065080) polymorphism is found to be associated with cold hypoalgesia, less heat, pin prick and mechanical hyperalgesia, whereas, 1103C>G (rs2222747) is associated with reduced cold hyaesthesia. None of the TRPV polymorphisms give impaired functions, suggesting its indirect linkage to pain *via* somatosensory abnormalities than direct function in pain [7]. In a complex manner, inflammatory mediator bradykinin enhances mechanical pain through Purinoreceptor 2X (P2X2,3) receptors mediation, and upregulates TRPV1 activation and Adenosine triphosphate (ATP) production *via* keratinocytes, Nerve growth factor (NGF) signaling *etc.*, thus causing mechanical hyperalgesia [8, 9]. However, inflammation induced hyperalgesia involves several other inflammatory mediators besides bradykinin alone [10].

Following the footprints of TRP gene family, Anoctamin 1(ANO1), a calcium activated chloride channel senses heat related pain detection. It depolarizes the neuron, causing generation of action potential. Animal studies confirmed its role in propagating heat stimuli, but not mechanical noxious stimuli by gene knockout, tail flick tests and chemical inhibition methods [11, 12].

Mechanical Pain

TRPV3 receptors mainly found in keratinocytes are activated by development of ATP by the cells. They are sensitized on moderate temperature ranges on repeated stimuli being found in traces in sensory neurons, as they are more associated with mechanical hyperalgesia. A polymorphic study shows the nominal association for TRPV3 gene SNP rs7217270 and TRPV1 gene SNP rs222741 with migraine related pain while no polymorphic study is found in TRPV2 [13].

TRPV4 channels are found abundantly in blood vessels, kidney cells *etc.* and act as sensors to mechanical, acidic and thermal pain. These channels promote inflammation and hyperalgesia on initiation as their murine knockouts show hypoalgesia in response to thermal, acidic and mechanical pain stimuli. Furthermore, TRPV4 knockout mice have longer latency to escape following hyperalgesia induced by inflammation in hot plate test [14].

Cold Pain

TRPA1 is sensitized at temperature below 18°C. Although being a cold sensor, due to their co-localization with TRPV1, cold stimuli related signals are misinterpreted as those from heat ones by a phenomenon named paradoxical cold [15]. Carriers of A allele in rs11988795 G>A SNP of TRPA1 glu/lys-179 polymorphism is associated with greater olfactory and cold related pain stimuli detection [16]. TRPA1 710>A (rs920829) polymorphism is also found to be associated with greater paradoxical heat sensation [7]. TRP channels induced cooling related pain signals are blocked by prostaglandin E2 receptors (PGE2) as shown in a cell culture study by decreasing cooling range from 32°C to 18°C causing reduced threshold for PKA values, thus, depicting an inhibitory effect of PGE2 on TRPM8 channel activation by cooling. In order to understand the genetic predictors of acute experimental cold and hot pain sensitivity in humans, Kim *et al.* investigated the role of TRPA1, TRPM8, TRPV1, opioid receptor delta 1 (OPRD1), catechol-o-methyltransferase (COMT) and Fatty acid amide hydrolase (FAAH) in four major ethnic populations. Haploblocks have been derived from the genes in European and American population, which are found to be associated more with females than males with respect to short duration cold pain sensitivity [17]. A dopamine active transporter 1 gene (DAT-1) or solute carrier family 6 member 3(SCL6A3) polymorphism study showed that carriers of homozygous 10-allele has enhanced cold associated pain tolerance than 9 allele carriers [18].

TRPM8 activates at low temperature as well as during inflammation. They co-express with Tropomyosin receptor kinase A TrkA (NGF receptors) and act *via* NGF signaling pathway, however, they do not produce heat induced hyperalgesia. Murine studies demonstrated that TRPM8 channel co expressed with GDNF family receptors, GFRα3 receptors and evokes heat hyperalgesia as well as cold responses in TRPM8 dependent manner [19]. Not until recently, it has been reported in a murine study that expression of TRPV1, TRPA1 and TRPM8 is controlled by a zinc- finger and BTB domain containing protein 20(ZBTB20), reduced expression of which hampers the activation of these channels in nociceptors [20]. While all the above given genes influence cold or heat pain stimuli to variable degrees, a sodium channel Na1.7 coded by sodium channel, voltage gated, type 9 alpha (SCN9A) is essential for transducing cold related signals. A study even highlighted rare A allele of rs6746030 association with higher pain values in various pain related conditions [21].

In contrary to the mechanism of TRP gene family, which detects and upregulates the pain related signals, Potassium channels subfamily K member 2 (KCNK2) are reported to act as antagonist to thermal stimuli *via* blocking bradykinin action, thus preventing inflammatory pain. In a murine knockout study, it is confirmed that KCNK2 deficient mice has ongoing heat transduction and inflammation induced pain [22]. Inhibition of KCNK2 channel causes activation of ANO1 channels *via* prostaglandins during inflammation.

Chemical Stimuli

For the detection of altered pH, TRPV1, acid sensing ion channel (ASIC) are found guilty [23]. ASIC1 are found to be responsible for generating afferent potential in case of low pH as well as inflammatory conditions as interplanter acidic saline in mice and humans cause pain, while ASIC3 is found to reduce inflammation in arthritic mice [24]. ASIC genes are found to be influencing agent in diseases like migraine [25]. ASIC is blocked by oxytocin and opioids so they may act as potential therapeutic target for analgesics [26].

Table 1. Genetic studies conducted on pain transduction.

PLACE	SAMPLE SIZE	GENE(S)	DISEASE	DIAGNOSIS	INFERENCE	AUTHORS
Japan	Subjects =355	P2X7 (rs1718125, rs2708092, rs1180012, rs208293, rs1718136, rs7132846)	Induced cold pain	Cold pressure induced pain, Fentanyl injection	Cold pressor test was significantly lower in subjects who carried homozygous haplotype (GTAAAC) in the P2RX7 gene compared with the other subjects.	[28]
USA	Subjects =735	TRP	Heat and cold pain	VAS, Haplotyping	Pain related haplotypes derived depicting TRP was associated with cold and heat related pain	[18]
Japan	Subjects =56	ASIC, VR-1	Proton or acid induced Pain	VAS, genotyping	High acidic conditions in blood activates ASIC causing pain, along with activation of VR-1 only in extreme acidic condition	[31]
UK	Subjects =33	ASIC	Pain	VAS, Ionotophoresis, Genotyping	ASIC activation causes pain, which is reduced by NSAIDs, irrespective of temperature, depicting a minor role of VR-1 in pH related pain	[32]
Belgium	Cases =21 Controls =33	IL-6	Fibro-myalgia	ACR-FM, Hamilton Depression Rating Scale (HDRS, Dolrimetery		[33]

(Table 1) contd.....

PLACE	SAMPLE SIZE	GENE(S)	DISEASE	DIAGNOSIS	INFERENCE	AUTHORS
UK	Cases =1098 Controls =3270	TRPV1 (rs8065080)	Osteoarth-ritis of Knee	VAS, Kellgren Lawrence scores	Ile-Ile genotype was associated with lower risk of osteoarthritis, reduced disease severity and lower pain scale readings	[34]
Germany	Subjects =81	TRPA1 (rs11988795)	Induced pain	VAS, Induced Heat, cold, pressure, chemical pain, olfactory and odor testing	TRPA1 gene minor allele A was associated with enhanced cold related pain stimuli and altered olfactory sensation.	[17]

Beside the peripheral nociception, there are set of subcutaneous receptors namely purinergic receptor X and Y (P2X and P2Y genes). P2X and P2Y gene families have a complex involvement in transduction of pain. Their activation *via* ATP generation through kerantinocytes enhances nociceptors. P2X3 receptors are found to be inducing inflammatory nociception by making primary afferent nociceptors more susceptible by interacting with TRPA1, 5-hydroxytryptamine (5-HT3) and 5-hydroxytryptamine 1alpha (5-HT1A) receptors [27]. Furthermore, haplotype based association study confirmed rs1718125 G>A polymorphism of P2X7 gene to be related with cold pain and a cold pain sensitivity alongwith reduced analgesia [28].

Inflammation induced nociception is observed to be mediated *via* TRPA1, 5-HT3 and 5-HT1A receptors. Furthermore, TRPM8 forms a complex with 5-HT receptors and phosopholipase D, thus reversing pain hypersensitivity [29]. Astonishingly, 5-HT or serotonin was involved in enhancing nociception at peripheral level as it gives analgesic effects in pain at central level. It acts *via* an indirect mechanism to activate sensory neurons through neutrophill migration, causing local release of dopamine, norepinephrine and prostaglandin causing inflammation mediated nociception and hyperalgesia, which is blocked by non-selective inhibitors of cyclooxygenase 2 (COX), beta 1,2 adrenergic receptors (ADRβ1,2) and dopamine proving involvement of multiple agents. However, 5-HT induced mechanical hyperalgesia is mediated by norepinephrine in dose dependent manner. A novel study on 5-HTRA1 SNP rs6295 polymorphism shows that carriers of minor A allele have low susceptibility to thermal pain stimuli [30].

2. CONDUCTION

Conduction involves conversion of numerous set of receptor potentials from the various sensory neurons, to form an action potential which transfers to the synaptic plate at the dorsal horn of spinal cord *via* secondary neurons. Once the receptor potential is generated, it requires a continuous and minimum threshold to propagate till synaptic level before submitting it ultimately to the higher brain regions.

Similar to ion channels present in transduction process, conduction also involves an array of ion channels. Hyperpolarization activated cyclic nucleotide gated cation channel (HCN) belongs to a class of channels that are permeable to both sodium and potassium ions, with four types; HCN1, 2, 3 and 4. They are essential for maintaining a continuous generation of action potential by acting as frequency modulators of continuous firing rate. It has been found that HCN2 channel influences firing rate in Nav1.8 expressing neurons [35]. A class of potassium channels KCNQ contributes remarkably in pain conduction. A member of KCNQ genes potassium voltage gated channel family member 4(kv3.4 or KCNC4) has been found to regulate action potential and firing rate following a spinal nerve injury in mice study. This has placed them in series of potential targets for drug delivery [36]. Another member of potassium channel sub-type is Kv9.1 channel encoded by KCNS1 gene that plays an anti-nociceptive role in pain conduction. It has been found that KCNS1 gene knockdowns demonstrate lowered pain thresholds and enhanced firing rates. Moreover, siRNA mediated knockdowns of kv9.1 gene demonstrate neuropathic pain behavior [37].

G-protein coupled inward rectifying potassium channels (GIRK) family is a potassium sensitive channel group with two subtypes; one expressing in brain and other in cardiac muscles. They are associated with opioid induced analgesia. A knockout study shows that GIRK channel activation, along with opioid receptor activation, inhibits nociceptive transmission thus leading to opioid induced analgesia [38]. KCNJ3 or GIRK1 knockout or chemical inhibition leads to elevated thermal nociception and blunted opioid derived analgesia. GIRK2 is essential for opioid induced peripheral analgesia and signaling [39]. Interestingly GIRK1 and GIRK 2 act at post synaptic level, quite different to all their siblings [40]. Brain type GIRK1,2 are activated by opioids as well as ethanol, giving opioid and ethanol induced analgesia which was confirmed by GRIK2 knockout study using weaver mice [41, 42].

The opening of GRIK channels is also found to reduce hyperalgesia in rat mussator muscles [43]. KCNJ6 or GIRK3 has been examined in several chronic pain conditions and it is inferred that A allele of rs2070995 is a potential risk allele as individuals homozygous for A allele require higher analgesic doses as compared to G allele [44, 45]. A distinct set of receptors namely nociception/ orphanin receptors work in conjunction with GIRK channels. Their activation causes GIRK channel sensitization in periaqueductal grey (PAG) area of brain [46]. Sodium channels (SC) is a family of sodium conducting ion channels. There are several members in this class including; SCN1A, SCN2A, SCN3A, SCN5A, SCN8A, SCN9A, SCN10A and SCN11A. However, not all of them are found relevant in pain studies. SCN1A or Nav1.1 is up regulated following a nerve injury, inducing neuropathic pain [47]. Surprisingly, auditory induced pain is found to be associated with $Na_v1.7$ while Nav1.6 is down regulated [48]. It has been documented that long term nerve injury causes altered gene expression in prefrontal cortex region in function of receptors such as N-methyl-D-aspartic acid (NMDA), SCN1A *etc.* shown by reverse transcriptase-quantitative PCR (RT-QPCR) [49].

SCN8A is located in nodes of Ranvier and at the initial segments. However, it has not been documented to be associated with pain. SCN9A or Nav1.6 is found to be associated with increased pain as well as mechanical cold allodynia [50]. It is inactivated by ankyrin-G protein directly as well as by channel clustering [51]. Their Knockouts have been reported to have reduced mechanical hyperalgesia. It owns a major part of muscle channelopathies [52]. Three genes SCN9A, SCN10A and SCN11A that encode sodium channels are observed in sensing neurons. SCN9A propagates action potentials as well as repair neuronal network of brain. SCN9A loss of function is associated with insensitivity to pain while gain of function causes channelopathies (*e.g.* paroxysmal extreme pain disorders).

SCN9A carriers, who have a defective $Na_v1.7$ remain pain free, which makes it a novel target for sodium selective drugs [53]. SCN10A ($Na_v1.8$) is a teradotoxin (TTX)-resistant sodium channel, found in nociceptors, is also significant contributor to pain conduction. Though, encoded channel $Na_v1.8$ does not induce action potential but plays a significant role in setting the pain thresholds. It induces hyperexcitability of neurons *via* TNF-α *via* p38MAPK dependent manner [54]. They are found to enhance muscle related pain when co expressed 5HT3A receptors in temporo-mandibular disorder(TMD) or myofacial pain states in gender specific manner where females are more vulnerable [55].Recently, a mutation R1279P is found in SCN9A, in limb pain patients, which induces hyper depolarization and enhanced firing rate [56]. SCN11A gets activated, close to the resting membrane potential and mutations in this gene have been associated to the loss of pain perception. Voltage gated sodium channel nociceptors specific SCN genes SCN1A, SCN3A, SCN8A, SCN9A, and SCN11A along with the potassium channels encoding KCNQ genes play a significant role in nociceptive conduction. Nav1.3 channels are associated with upregulation of pain related signaling in response to spinal nerve injury and an altered mRNAs profile in dorsal horn neurons during pain conditions. They hyper sensitize and leads to activation of ATP evoked P2X3 receptor mediated depolarization of nociceptive neurons that in turn is modulated by protein kinase C [57].

P2 receptors are associated with excitatory or pre-nociceptive function at peripheral level while anti-nociceptive function at central level *e.g.* P2X3. P2X3 transmits pain signals by facilitating glutamate release. They are seen during nerve injury [58]. P2X7 receptors activation causes upregulation of nociceptive signaling. Being expressed during inflammation, they cause thermal hyperalgesia [59]. Bradykinin produced by BK gene is the key element to detect and propagate mechanical, heat and inflammation induced pain signals. It is known to sensitize TRPV1, TRP1 and protein kinase C. In clinical trial studies, selective bradykinin1 receptor antagonist administration reverses the inflammatory and mechanical hyperalgesia by desensitization of peripheral and spinal neurons [60]. They are even found to activate ANO1 channel while inhibiting M-type potassium channels, thus promoting increased depolarization and action potential firing rate [61]. It has been confirmed that ANO1 knockouts show a reduced thermal pain and inflammation induced hyperalgesia [12].

A class of molecules named interleukins is secreted during inflammation. They are highly associated with increasing pain levels by propagating signal conduction. They are found to be in elevated amount, especially in case of diseases involving inflammation such as rheumatoid arthritis. Several polymorphic studies have highlighted specific diseases susceptibility related to a particular genotype. T allele of rs1800587 in interleukin 1(IL-1α) gene was found to be associated with higher risk of developing disc degeneration and related back pain [62]. A similar finding in IL-4 gene has been observed, where minor allele rs1805010 is associated with enhanced radiologically visible degeneration and T17 helper (th17) cell proliferation [63]. Many other polymorphisms such as G allele of rs3811047 of interleukin 7 (IL-7) gene are found to be associated with disease severity [64, 65].

Calcitonin gene related peptide (CGRP) is involved in inflammatory pain. It is expressed in keratinocytes and causes functional changes in them causing proliferation and cytokine production, thus raising pain levels [66].

Glial cell derived growth factor (GDNF) are found to promote neuronal growth. They also have disputed modulatory function in both conduction as well as inhibition of pain signals. GDNF inhibits pain transmission pre-synaptically [67]. Alpha 2C adrenergic receptors (ADRA2C) are required to maintain continuous signaling till presynaptic level. A specific DRA2C 322-325 deletion variant has been studied in relation to pain perception, where ADRA2C Del homozygotes are found to possess higher pain score in relation to various painful stimuli [68]. Angiotensin converting enzyme (ACE) is responsible for increasing the blood pressure by altering fluid volumes and pressures. Elevated levels of ACE are found in various inflammatory pain conditions such as rheumatoid arthritis, osteoarthritis and ankylosing spondylosis. ACE I/D polymorphism has been examined in the above conditions with an outcome of D allele carriers, especially DD homozygotes being at the highest risk of developing these conditions [69 - 71].

Table 2. Genetic studies conducted on conduction of pain.

PLACE	SAMPLE SIZE	GENE(S)	DISEASE	DIAGNOSIS	INFERENCE	AUTHORS
Finland	Subjects =181	IL-1α	Low back pain	Questionnaire, MRI	Carriers of the IL-1RNA(1812) allele had an increased risk of low back pain and carriers of this allele in combination with the IL-1alphaT(889) or IL-1betaT(3954) allele had a higher risk of low back pain occurrence and higher pain intensity than non-carriers.	[72]
Norway	Cases=121	IL-1α (rs1800587)	Lumbar radicular pain due to disc herniation	VAS, Pressure Pain Thresholds	IL-1α CT/TT genotype rs1800587 may be associated with increased pain intensity and corresponding reduced PPT during the first year after disk herniation.	[61]
Spain	Cases=50 Controls =129	Il-1α,β eNOS, TNF, iNOS	Lumbar disc hernia	MRI, Genotyping	Carriers of the CC genotype of the IL-1β (+3953 T/C) SNP were more frequent among Lumbar disc hernia(LDH) patients suggesting some potential role of the IL-1β SNP on LDH pathogenesis. The eNOS (-786 T/C) and iNOS (22 G/A) SNPs were more frequent among the control subjects, suggesting their possible protective role against LDH.	[73]
Germany	Cases= 90 Controls=39	IL4R (rs1805010)	Rheumatoid arthritis	Disease Activity Score, ELISA, Flowcytometry, Genotyping	Minor allele contributes to increased Th17 cell frequency, enhanced clinical activity, and accelerated radiographic progression in RA by rendering CD4 T cells from RA patients insensitive to the attenuating effect of IL-4 on Th17 cell development.	[63]
Canada	Cases=181	IL-6, IL-10, TGF-1β	Juvenile rheumatoid arthritis	Childhood Health Assessment Questionnaire (CHAQ), visual analogue scale physician's global assessment of disease activity (PGA)	he correlation of IL-6 genotype with pain and the possible association of the TGF-beta1 codon 25 genotype with short-term radiographic damage (G/C with greater risk and G/G with decreased risk) suggests that both these polymorphisms may be useful early prognostic indicators	[74]
China	Cases =276 Controls =276	IL-7 (rs3811047)	Rheumatoid arthritis	Joint swelling index Resting pain, ACR-diagnosis, Genotyping	G allele of rs3811047 has certain influence on the condition of RA patients with higher pain ratings, however no notable difference found in overall population	[75]
Sweden	Cases =35 Controls=25	IL-12, MIP-α, β, CRP	Shoulder pain, Neck pain	standard Nordic questionnaire for analysis of musculoskeletal symptoms, Borg scale	Higher levels of major intrinsic protein alpha (MIP-α, β), IL-12 were found significantly high in expression in individuals with neck/shoulder pain than other ILs or CRP	[76]
USA	Cases= 150	IL-12	Fibromyalgia	American college of rheumatology criteria for FM, Whole genome sequencing	Patients with ZNF77 mutations have high IL-12 levels, causing more inflammatory pain	[77]
Denmark	Cases= 281	CRP	Osteoarthritis of the knee	Kellgren/ Lawrence scale Pressure pain thresholds temporal summation of pain, and conditioning pain modulation Biochemical tests	Higher serum matrix metalloproteinase (MMP)-mediated breakdown of CRP levels were associated with more central sensitization, and seen more profoundly in women.	[78]
USA	Subjects =72	BDNF	Placebo induced pain	PET, (VAS), Genotyping	BDNF rs6265 (val/val) genotype is more active in reward system in stress to compensate pain.	[79]
USA	Cases =95 Controls =58	BDNF	Fibromyalgia	VAS, Fibromyalgia impact questionnaire (RIQ), ELISA, IJR	BDNF val/val genotype has high levels high sensitivity CRP levels and BMI in fibromyalgia patients than in normal individuals. However no significant associations could be found in pain scores.	[80]

(Table 2) contd.....

PLACE	SAMPLE SIZE	GENE(S)	DISEASE	DIAGNOSIS	INFERENCE	AUTHORS
Brazil	Cases =30 Controls =30	BDNF	Fibromyalgia	Immuno-assay, HAM-D	Increased levels of BDNF were found in Fibromyalgia patients as compared to normal individuals irrespective of depression levels. But no relation could be derived with pain scores	[81]
Denmark, Finland	Cases: Osteo Arthritis =578 Sciatia =195 Amputed=100	SCN9A (rs6746030)	Osteoarthritis Sciatica Post-amputation Discotomy	WOMAC scale, VAS	The rare Aallele is associated with high pain score in SNP rs6746030 among OA and sciatia patients.	[82]
China	Cases =200	SCN9A (3312G>T)	Post-operative pain	VAS, Pain tolerance and threshold, Placebo analgesic	SCN9A 3312 T allele is associated with low pain perception, leading to reduced analgesic requirement postoperatively	[83]
Germany	Subjects =75	SCN9A (rs4126863 and rs6746030)	Pain stimuli response	Bioelectric test, Genotyping	Reduced olfaction and reduced nociception are correlated by SCN9A haplotype	[84]
China	Cases =69 Controls =102	SCN11A	Episodic pain	Pedigree analysis, Haplotyping	SCN11A C673C>T, C2423C>G showed co segregation in families, which were not detected in normal individuals. It causes increased gain of function in SCN11A with lower pain thresholds and high firing rate of signals	[85]
Israel Finland	Lumber pain =151 Amputation =199 Sciatia=195 Controls=185	KCNS1 (rs734784)	Low back pain Limb amputation	VAS, Genotyping, immune-assay, RT-PCR	KCNS1 allele for rs734784 is prognostic risk indicator for chronic pain (coding for valine) rs13043825 is also found to be significantly associated with high pain scores	[86]
USA	OA=311 CLBP=75 Controls=63	KCNJ3, KCNJ6	Chronic low back pain, Knee replacement	Postsurgical pain scale, VAS, Ischemic tourniquet pain test, GIRK Related Risk Score, Genotyping	Polymorphism in KCNJ6 gene was related to high pain scores depicting more vulnerability to pain.	[87]
Germany	Subjects =16	PGE2	Inflammation and trauma induced pain	Clinical trial proton induced pain Questionare	During acidic conditions, PGE2 can initiate nociceptors activation by protons present in skin and muscle	[88]
Norway	Cases =93	IL1A, IL18RAP, IL18R1, MMP3	Chronic low backache, Lumber disc degeneration	Oswestry disability scale, VAS, MRI, CT scans	IL18RAP polymorphism (rs1420100) was associated with severe, multiple disc degeneration. rs917997 and rs1420106 were associated with post treatment improvement in disability. Haplotype association analysis of 5 SNPs spanning across IL18RAP, IL18R1 and IL1A genes revealed significant associations with improvement in disability and reduction in pain..	[89]
Finland	Cases =155 Controls =179	IL-6,IL1A, IL1B, IL1RN, TNFA, IL2, IL4, IL4R, IL10, IFNG	Inter-vertebral disc disease	Genotyping	Haplotype GGGA for the four IL-6 SNPs were found more frequently in patients than normal subject and were associated with attribute risk for the disc related pain.	[90]
Turkey	Cases =221 Controls =200	ACE I/D) MTHFR (C677T)	osteoarthritis	Kellgren-Lawrence Grade, Lequesnes' functional index, VAS	DD allele in ACE and CC genotype in MTHFR was found to be related with higher occurrence of osteoarthritis and high pain scores	[71]
Turkey	Cases =138 Controls =71	GSTM1, GSTT1, GSTP1-ILE105VAL and ACE	Ankylosing spondylitis	Bath Ankylosing Spondylitis Activity Index, the Bath Ankylosing Spondylitis Metrology Index, Bath Ankylosing Spondylitis Functional Index, Numeric rating scale	Significantly higher levels of CRP and the NRS pain scores in the patients with ACE ID or DD genotypes compared to those in the patients with ACE II genotypes. The present results showed that genes involved in protection from oxidative stress and ACE gene may influence disease development and course in AS.	[91]

(Table 2) contd.....

PLACE	SAMPLE SIZE	GENE(S)	DISEASE	DIAGNOSIS	INFERENCE	AUTHORS
USA	Controls=73 (Caucasian=37 African=36)	ADRA2C Ins/del	Pain perception	VAS, digit symbol substitution test, cold presser test, clinical drug trials	ADRA2C (dele/de)l homozygotes had higher pain scores in response to cold than heterozygotes. Their reading improved after α-2 agonist proving more ADRA2C causes more pain relief	[68]
USA	Cases =21 Controls =25	ADRA2C	Chronic low back pain	Clinical trial, Baroreflex sensitivity test	Hypoalgesia due to ADRA2C antagonist was less significant in CLBP subjects causing no anti-nociception during baroreflex tests.	[92]
USA	Controls =39	GCH1 (rs8007267, rs3783641, rs8007201, rs4411417, rs752688)	Capsaicin related pain	Clinical drug trial, PET scanning, Visual analogue scale, Genotyping	GCH1 gene polymorphism was related to lower pain ratings.	[93]

3. TRANSMISSION

Once the action potential has reached the presynaptic level, various ions channels enter the scene, as their opening or closing decides the fate of signal, whether the signal will be transmitted and with what amplitude. On reaching the presynaptic level, calcium channels open generating a presynaptic potential; leading to the release of various neurotransmitters especially acetylcholine in synaptic cleft. From there the signal is transmitted to the higher corticals of the brain and spinal cord. However, several neurotransmitters such as Gamma- Aminobutyric acid (GABA), dopamine, glutamate and acetylcholine alongwith a variety of receptors such as opioid receptor, cannaboid family members and many others also play significant role in transmission of pain signals.

Table 3. Genetic studies conducted on transmission of pain

PLACE	SAMPLE SIZE	GENE(S)	DISEASE	DIAGNOSIS	INFERENCE	AUTHORS
USA	Cases =290	GABAAβ1	Low back pain, Sciatic disc Degenerative disc disease	Short form-36, Movement impairment subscale of Roland Morris scale	Haplotype in GABAa-β1 unit may act as endogenous muscle relaxant for SNPs (rs4694846, rs17461905,rs6813436, rs7439087, rs6290)	[113]

(Table 3) contd.....

PLACE	SAMPLE SIZE	GENE(S)	DISEASE	DIAGNOSIS	INFERENCE	AUTHORS
Israel	Subjects=192	MAO-A, DRD4, SLC6A3	Induced cold pain	Heat/ cold stimuli thresholds, Genotyping	Low dopaminergic activity can be associated with high pain sensitivity and vice versa. Further, 10 and 11 allele of SCL6A3were associated with less cold pain tolerance than 9 or 4 allele.	[100]
Israel	Subjects= 105	SLC6A3 (3-UTR 40-bp VNTR)	Induced Cold pain	Clinical drug trial, Heat/ cold stimuli thresholds, Numerical pain scale	Subjects with two copies of the 10-allele showed significantly greater tolerance than the 9-allele homozygote carriers and the heterozygote carriers in comparison to the placebo.	[19]
Taiwan	Subjects=72	OPRM1 (IVS2+31G>A), OPRK1, OPRD1	Pressure pain sensitivity	Heat/ cold pain stimuli thresholds, Beck Anxiety Inventory, Genotyping	The Pressure pain threshold, in subjects with the minor allele A of the IVS2+31G>A polymorphism of the OPRM1 gene was significantly higher than those with major allele G. Neither pressure pain threshold nor tolerance between major and minor alleles of other SNPs of the OPRM1, OPRK1, and OPRD1 genes were significantly different.	[110]
USA	Subjects=167	OPRM1 (A118G)	Pressure pain sensitivity	Heat/cold stimuli thresholds Genotyping	Rare allele of OPRM1 (A118G) was associated with pain in sex specific manner showing higher thresholds in men and its presence showed the vice versa in females	[114]
Taiwan	Cases =120	OPRM1-(A118G)	Osteoarthritis	Clinical drug trial, VAS, Genotyping	Patients with AA genotype showed greater improvements post operatively, requiring far less amount of morphine than AG or AA individuals	[115]

(Table 3) contd.....

PLACE	SAMPLE SIZE	GENE(S)	DISEASE	DIAGNOSIS	INFERENCE	AUTHORS
Sweden	Cases =80 Controls=56	OPRM1-(A118G) CACNAD2 (rs5030977) ABCB1 (C3435T) (rs1045642)	Low back pain	Clinical drug trial, VAS, EORTC-OLQ-30 form, Radioimmunoassay	Control group had higher levels of β-endorphins. Major allele for CACNAD2 and minor allele of OPRM1 were associated with increased opioid sensitivity.	[98]
Denmark	Subjects=33	OPRM1 ABCB1	Human experimental pain	Heat/ cold/ electrical pain stimuli thresholds Electrical nerve stimulation	G allele of OPRM1 is associated with reduced antinociceptive effect. The combined wild-type genotype 3435CC-2677GG was associated with less anti-nociceptive effect of oxycodone than the carriers of the variant alleles.	[116]

Glutamate is an essential component for pain signal transmission. A class of glutamate receptor family gene GRIN1 has been studied in relation to pain and it is reported to be up regulated during inflammatory pain condition such as tendinitis along with N-methyl-D-aspartate (NMDA) receptors and substance P [94, 95]. Acetylcholine is the most crucial component in synaptic transmission. Although acetylcholine is a neurotransmitter but acts in two distinct ways, either propagates or diminishes the pain signal. It has been found that acetylcholine injections are found to reduce pain. Contrarily, acetylcholine released at the site of injury tendinitis causes elevated levels of pain, leading to inflammation [96, 97]. Genes coding for voltage dependent calcium channel subunit alpha-2/ delta-1(CACNA2D1) controls the influx of ions to produce membrane depolarization. In a Swedish study, it has been inferred that presence of major allele G is associated with higher opioid sensitivity [98]. These channels are of high therapeutic relevance as they are the targets of pregabalin and gabapentin (GABA inhibiting drugs) [99]. Pain has been described by neuroscientists as a subjective emotion. Hence, an ample share of pain modulation is accommodated by dopaminergic or catelocholenergic neurotransmitters. Dopamine has been found to be related to pain in a reverse manner [100]. Lower dopamine levels are associated with pain related symptoms in neurodegenerative disease like Parkinson disease. Concordant to the existing thought, recently it has been found in a murine study that dopamine receptor D2 (DRD2) agonists could treat mechano-nociception but fail to cure thermal nociception [101]. There are contradictory evidences in other pain conditions such as fibromyalgia, where no relation has been found in FM subjects showing an altered dopaminergic mechanism involved in fibromyalgia [102].

Adrenergic hormones mainly serotonin, adrenaline and nor-adrenaline and their respective receptors influence the pain at spinal and supraspinal levels. Their reuptake inhibitors attenuate pain by preventing their absorption at synapses, causing increased postsynaptic monoamines and sustained descending pathway activity [103]. While the activity of dopamine and serotonin are variable, providing both nociceptive as well as antinociceptive behavior, the noradrenaline shows a purely antinociceptive effect. Therefore, selective noradrenaline reuptake inhibitors provide more robust antinociceptive effects than those of serotonin reuptake inhibitors. Several pain conditions such as osteoarthritis and rheumatoid arthritis involve disease worsening, with loss of noradrenalinergic fibers in synovial tissue [104, 105]. However, higher levels of noradrenaline in cerebrospinal fluid preoperatively are related to greater pain scores [106]. A polymorphism has been studied in ADRA2C gene where del/del homozygotes have higher pain scores in response to cold than heterozygotes. Their reading improved after α-2 agonist proving more ADRA2C causes more pain relief [68]. Glucocorticoids work in synergy with adrenaline. Patients with rheumatoid arthritis have been tested with the hormone therapy for pain management. However, results vary due to individual cortisol sensitivity variation [107, 108].

GABA receptors are the major G protein coupled receptors. They are the key elements in pain transmission as glutamate being a major transporting agent across the synaptic cleft. Activation of GABA-β receptor induces presynaptic inhibition of decreasing presynaptic glutamate release [109]. A class of μ-opioid receptors 1(OPRM1) is found to be associated with analgesic requirement in a dose dependent manner. The minor allele G (IVS2+31G>A) is found to be related to higher pain rating, more profoundly in women [110]. In two other studies, this polymorphism is also found to be related to pressure pain sensitivity and slow recovery in posttraumatic or post-operative conditions [111, 112].

4. MODULATION

Modulation involves a huge range of effects on pain perception which may either be increasing it or attenuating it. However, both the contrasting mechanism involves descending pain pathway with distinct key players planning the fate of pain, *i.e.*, whether to suppress it or to enhance it. Pain modulation may occur at three levels; peripheral level, dorsal level of spinal cord and at higher corticals of brain. At periphery, most of the TRPA, TRPV and ASIC ion channels are known to upregulate stimuli specific signals. The signals generated by them are eventually conducted by SCN sodium channels and HCN channels. Calcium channels further maintain the signal intensity presynaptically. On the contrary, potassium channels are known to work as anti nociceptive.

The activation of P2 family genes causes activation of various surface receptors, such as P2X4,7 which are responsible for upregulating several inflammatory mediators, leading to hyperalgesia. Specific polymorphisms found in these genes may upregulate the pain. P2X3 receptors show dual effect like opioid receptors as they act pre-nociceptive at peripheral level while anti-nociceptive at central level, thus reducing pain [58]. Opioid receptors mediate pain in conjugation with P2X3 receptors *via* phospholipase C (PLC) dependent pathways [117]. Purinergic receptor (P2Y12) decreases inflammatory and neuropathic pain by blocking production of cytokines and thermal pain sensitization through IL-7 receptor mediation pathway. Suppression of these receptors has shown to give relief from pain [118, 119]. KCNJ6 channel polymorphism is associated with post operative pain [38]. Neuropeptide Y modulates pain at peripheral level *via* blocking signaling caused by substance P at dorsal horn level as well as causing an anti-hyperalgesic effect [120]. TRP1 secrete substance P *via* inflammatory mediator CGRP thus upregulating the pain. CGRP is also upregulated by prostaglandins during inflammatory pain conditions, hence administration of specific COX inhibitors wipe away pain [121]. As per the universal norm, once the primary receptor potential is generated and if the whole is accompanied by inflammation, it will certainly end up regulating the pain. It has been inferred from several studies that in many inflammatory pain conditions, the primary receptor potential is amplified by inflammatory mediators, thus causing generation of an enhanced pain receptor potential [10]. Here variable forms of such agents such as interleukins give a profound regulatory effect. Various other inflammatory mediators such as interleukins, cytokines and bradykinin come into scene, intensifying the whole scenario of pain realization. It involves activation of Protein kinase C (PKC), mitogen activated protein kinase (p38) and 9-Jun-N-terminal kinase (JNK) as well. Synthesis of IL-1β, IL-6 and TNF is associated with upregulation of bradykinin B1, B2 receptors [122]. Thus selective bradykinin -1 receptor antagonists have shown to reverse inflammatory and mechanical hyperalgesia by desensitization of peripheral and spinal neurons.

Various vascular factors such as VEGF contribute to pain modulation as various polymorphic variations in these genes alter the pain signaling properties [123]. There are various neurotransmitter genes and receptors that influence pain at synaptic and dorsal level. Serotonin acts both at peripheral and cortical level in contradicting manner, being pro-nociceptive at periphery and anti-nociceptive at higher levels. Serotonin stored in platelets affects the process as higher serotonin causes upregulation of inflammatory mediators such as prostaglandins [124], serotonin causes nociception *via* neutrophil migration and local release of prostaglandins, dopamine and noradrenaline. Spinal cord injection of serotonin agonist causes dose dependent nociception which are reduced following administration of their antagonists [125]. Genetic studies reveal that the carriers of long allele have higher magnitude of pain ratings than those of short one [126]. Another study confirms that serotonin antagonists reduce the pain [127]. 5-Hydroxytryptamine receptor 3B gene HTR3B SNP (rs117644) has high Pain Catastrophising Score (PCS) values in T allele depicting cause of pain catestrophising due to anxiety and depression [128]. Similarly T allele of HTR2A (rs12584920) is part of risk regions for chronic widespread pain [129].

Serotonin is known to co-activate dopamine and noradrenaline neurotransmitters as well. Hence, Dopamine holds a significant value when it comes to pain modulation. It has been shown to act in *vice versa* manner in controlling pain which means lack of dopamine causes more pain. Hence, dopamine once released activates dopamine receptor D1 (DRD1) and adrenergic receptor beta1 (ADRβ1).

Serotonin, if injected intravenously, produces dose dependent hyperalgesia in mice, which is reduced by non selective COX, DRD or ADR receptor blockers, showing their role in pain modulation in synchronization [130]. Opioid and GABA receptor plays significant role at receptor level. As mentioned earlier, GABA blockage causes pain inhibition. However, its functions differ pre and post-synaptically. The postsynaptic transmission is mediated *via* activation of G protein coupled GRIK channels. So it is found that blockage of these channels largely prevents post synaptic membrane potential. So GABA plays differentially as presynaptic inhibition causes K^+ insensitivity while the postsynaptic inhibition causes K^+ sensitivity [109]. Opioid and cannaboid receptors comprise natural analgesic system of body. In dorsal root ganglion deltoid opioid receptors are present in lower levels on cell surface, in contrast to higher levels of intracellular receptors that are mainly associated with vesicles containing CGRP. Opioid receptor delta1 (OPRD1) activation leads to calcium influx which causes CGRP release. Hence, it has been observed that inflammatory pain may be treated with selective OPRD1 antagonists [131].

There are major differences found in pain perception rating between male and females in both human and animal based studies. In humans, it is found that men are less prone to pain or have a greater endurance due to protective mechanism of male androgenic hormone testosterone than women. A meta-analysis on female estrogen receptor gene, ER-α reveals that A allele of SNP rs9340799 is found to be having higher risk values in occurrence of osteoarthritis [132]. At cortical level, catechol-o-methyltransferase produced by COMT gene has emerged as a benchmark for pain perception in various populations across the globe. A specific nucleotide polymorphism has been examined and it is found that M allele of rs4680 SNP is associated with higher pain rating on various scales. Individuals with MM genotype had more pain, followed by VM and VV, in various diseases such as fibromyalgia, osteoarthritis and so on. In many studies, other SNPs of COMT gene such as rs4633, rs4818, and rs6269 constitute pain haplotypes [133].

Besides neurotransmitters, there are other several notable transporter genes which are found to be associated with pain perception and modulation. The lipid transporter gene apolipoprotein E (APOE) is a tri-allelic gene. Its E2 allele is found to be associated with higher disease susceptibility in migraine and fibromyalgia [134 - 136]. Similarly, P-glycoprotein gene family member ABCB1 (3435 C>T) is associated with lower morphine requirements in severe pain conditions [137]. The metabolic enzyme CYP2D6 also shows relevance to pain as reduced enzyme activity corresponds to reduced pain levels [138].

Table 4. Genetic studies conducted on modulation of pain.

PLACE	SAMPLE SIZE	GENE (S)	DISEASE	DIAGNOSIS	INFERENCE	AUTHORS
Denmark	Subjects =30	HTR3B	Inflammatory Pain	Pain catastrophising scales (PCS), Beck depression inventory scale (BDI), Speilberger stat trait anxiety inventory (STAI), Genotyping	T allele of rs117644 has high PCS values leading to catestrophising due to anxiety and depression	[128]
USA	Subjects =42	FAAH	Induced Pain	PANAS, POMS-TMD, Mcgill Pain Questionare, VAS, PET, Genotyping	FAAH Pro129/Pro129 homozygotes, reported greater placebo-induced μ-opioid, but not D2/3 dopaminergic, enhancements in neurotransmission.	[139]
USA/ Israel	Subjects =191	5HTTPR	Thermal pain	Genotyping	Carriers of long allele have high magnitude of pain perception than that of short allele of serotonin receptors	[126]
Sweden	Subjects =44	5HT3	Thermal induced pain	VAS Thermal grill illusion STAI Beck depression inventory (BDI)	Low HT expression is related to low thermal pain threshold values in normal. low 5-HTT is a risk factor for chronic pain states as well as for depression.	[140]
UK	Cases =164 Controls =172	HTR2A, TPH2	Chronic widespread pain	American college for rheumatology for FM, BDI	6 SNPs in HTR2A represents a risk region for Chronic Widespread Pain. while rs17289394 in TPH2 gene adds in increased pain levels and number of sites	[129]
Israel	Subjects =191	HTTLPR DRD4	Cold and conditional pain	Genotyping	No association found between pain and DRD4 polymorphism, but long allele for HTTLPR found to be having higher pain thresholds than short allele carrying individuals	[126]
Germany	Controls =33	GCH1, BHH, iNOS	Pain hyperalgesia,, Thermal pain	VAS, Electrical pain intensity test, Thermal pain tests	Less GCH function causes less pain. Decreased GCH1 function due to polymorphism acts against pain, giving pain protective haplotype for GCH1.	[141]
UK	Cases =164 Controls =172	SERPINA6, MC2R, CRH, CRHBP, CRHR1, POMC, NR3C1	Chronic widespread pain	Manchester coding system, Hospital Anxiety and depression (HAD) scale, General Health Questionnaire, Estimation of Sleep Problems Scale	Minor T allele of rs941601 of SERPINA6 gene and common A allele of rs8022616 are associated with severe pain	[142]
UK	Cases =197 Controls =197	GCH1 (rs10483639, rs3783641, rs8007267), OPRM1 (rs1777971, rs563649)	Chronic widespread pain	Genotyping	There was no association found between diseased and pain free subjects. So study failed to replicate previous pain protective haploypte in GCH1 and OPRM1	[143]
Romania	Cases=43	VEGF, HGF	Limb ischemia	Ankle brachial index	Insertion of VEGF/HGF reduces pain upto 65%	[123]
Canada	Cases =36 Controls =37	DRD3, COMT	Fibromyalgia	Cold and hot pain test, Genotyping	DRD3 (Ser9Gly) polymorphism influences Diffused Noxious Inhibitory Control efficacy and Thermal Pain No relationship was found between thermal pain and COMT	[144]

(Table 4) contd.....

PLACE	SAMPLE SIZE	GENE (S)	DISEASE	DIAGNOSIS	INFERENCE	AUTHORS
China	Cases =84 Controls =168	DRD4 (-521C/T)	Cold pain	Genotyping	TT genotype (C-521T) individuals have far low pain thresholds than CT or CC genotypes and enhanced opioid dependency	[145]
Italy	Cases=74	COMT (rs4680)	Chronic back pain Headache	Clinical drug trial Genotyping	Subjects with met/met genotype showed poor response to opioid analgesics as compared to other twos posing met/met genotype to a risk factor for pain	[146]
Poland	Cases =176	COMT (rs4680, rs4633, rs6269, rs4818)	Back pain Disc hernia	VAS for leg and back pain Oswestry disability index CT scans, MRI	COMT haplotype (A-C-C-G) associated with low metabolic activity of enzyme and showed better clinical results by ODI score and VAS score 1 year after surgery	[133]
Switzerland	Cases =137 Controls =99	COMT (rs4680)	Fibromyalgia	nociceptive flexion reflex, Quality of life and distress questionnaires	Met/met individuals showed higher central sensitization and higher distress levels than other two genotypes and controls	[147]
Spain	Cases =100	COMT (rs4680)	Fibromyalgia	ACR-FMS, Numerical rating scale, Hospital Anxiety and Depression Scale, Fibromyalgia Impact Questionnaire	Met/met genotype was associated with high pain perception, disability, anxiety and depression but not related with pressure pain levels	[148]
Norway	Cases =93	COMT (rs4680, rs4633)	Low back pain	VAS, Oswestry disability index	rs4680 and rs4633 were found to be associated with pain, anxiety and depression. The heterozygote individuals showed better analgesic effects than homozygous individuals	[149]
China	Subjects =200	COMT(rs6269, rs4633, rs4818, rs165599, rs4680)	Induced pain	Bioelectrical test, VAS	The haplotypes generated for these SNPs (rs6269, rs4633, rs4818, rs165599, and rs4680) were not found to be associated with pain perception in Chinese men.	[150]
Spain	Cases =113 Control =65	COMT (rs6269, rs4633, rs4818, rs4680)	Fibromyalgia	Bioelectrical nerve reflex test, Genotyping	FM patients were more sensitive to experimental pain than healthy volunteers and, in particular, FM individuals with the met/met genotype	[151]
Norway	Cases =1004	COMT, ADRB2	Chronic low back pain Neck pain	VAS, questionnaire, genotyping	Minor allele of rs2053044 SNP of ADRB2 gene was found to have higher chronic widespread pain and more pain areas.	[152]
USA	Cases =45	COMT (rs4680)	Fibromyalgia	Numerical rating scale, Coping Strategies Questionnaire, Pain Vigilance and Awareness Questionnaire	FM patients with the homozygous met/met genotype showed more pain	[153]
Brazil	Cases =51 Controls =51	COMT (rs4680) 5HT2A	Fibromyalgia	ACR-FM, Self made questionnaire	HT2A showed no relation with fibromyalgia while met/met carriers were found more prevalent in patients with fibromyalgia	[154]
Brazil	Cases =112 Controls =110	COMT(rs4680, rs4633)	Fibromyalgia	ACR-FM, Fibromyalgia Impact Questionnaire	Homozygous AA for rs4680 and CC for rs4633 were found to be associated with fibromyalgia and pain in about one third of FM patients.	[155]
Netherlands	Cases =78 Controls =37	COMT (rs4680), BDNF- (rs6265), OPRM1- A(118)G	Chronic low back pain	Electrical stimuli test, EEG	COMT Met allele and the BDNF Met allele augmented cortical pain processing, while reducing pain processing in pain-free controls. No significant effects were found concerning the OPRM1 A(118)G polymorphism	[156]
USA	Cases =69	COMT (rs6269, rs4633, rs4818, rs4680)	Lumbar disc degenerative disease	Oswestry Disability Index VAS for LBP	Haplotype analysis of four COMT SNPs, rs6269, rs4633, rs4818, and rs4680, also identified a common haplotype "ATCA" was associated with greater improvement in ODI	[157]

(Table 4) contd.....

PLACE	SAMPLE SIZE	GENE (S)	DISEASE	DIAGNOSIS	INFERENCE	AUTHORS
UK	Cases =1958	COMT ADRB2 SNPs (rs12654778, rs1042713)	Chronic widespread pain		Common functional ADRB2 haplotype combinations were associated with pain status and with both extent and duration of pain There were no associations of either CWP or pain status with COMT genotypes or haplotypes.	[158]
Israel	Cases =209 Controls =152	COMT (rs4680)	Fibromyalgia	ACR-RM	Met/met carriers were found to be more frequent in FM patients with increased sensitivity to pain while the majority of normal subjects lack Met allele	[159]
USA	Cases =89	COMT (rs6269, rs4633, rs4818, rs4680)	Neck pain	numeric rating scale VAS Michigan Critical Events Perception Scale	high pain sensitivity haplotype (A-C-C-G) was found to be associated with high pain ratings, slow recovery and enhanced distress symptoms	[160]
USA	Subjects =204	COMT (rs6269, rs4633, rs4818, rs4680, rs2097903 and rs6269)	Temporo-mandibular disorder	Numeric rating scale, Thermal pain thresholds	Subjects homozygous for the G-C-G-G haplotype experienced least pain as compared to other two genotypes	[161]
USA	Subjects =63	COMT (rs6269, rs4633, rs4818, rs4680)	Shoulder pain	Fear of Pain Questionnaire (FPQ-III), Catastrophizing Scale (PCS), VAS, Maximum voluntary isometric contraction (MVIC)	Low enzyme activity genotypes met/Met) and haplotypes were associated with higher pain rating and pain Catastrophizing	[162]
Mexico/ Spain	Cases: Mexicans =57 Spanish =78 Controls: Mexicans =33 Spanish =80	COMT rs2097903, rs6269, rs4633, rs4818, rs4680 and rs165599)	Fibromyalgia	Fibromyalgia Impact Questionnaire	In Spanish patients, there was a significant association of three SNPs (rs6269, rs4818, and rs4680) with FM than healthy controls, showing a more severe relation of 'high pain sensitivity' haplotype (ACCG) with FM. Mexican patients displayed weak association.	[163]
Sweden	Subjects =43	COMT (rs4680)	Induced pain	Clinical trial, Thermal pain thresholds, VAS	Met/met individuals showed higher pain rating than others and on administration of opioid drug the same group showed higher opioid induced hyperalgesia than other two groups	[164]
Turkey	Cases =379 Controls =290	COMT (rs4680)	Fibromyalgia	Algometry, FMS Impact Questionnaire score	Met/met subjects were found more in FMS patients than in controls. pain sensitivity scores were also higher in met/met genotypes than val/met or val/val genotypes	[165]
USA	Cases =69	COMT (rs6269, rs4633, rs4818, rs4680)	Degenerative disc disease	Oswestry Disability Index (ODI) visual analog score (VAS)	T allele for rs4633 was associated with improved ODI scores after surgery. The greatest mean improvement was found in SNPs, rs6269, rs4633, rs4818, and rs4680, based haplotype "ATCA"	[166]
USA	Cases =200 Controls =198	COMT (rs2097603, rs6269, rs4633, rs4818, rs4680)	Temporo-Mandibular Disorder	Quantitative Sensory Testing, Pressure algometry testing	The haplotype coding for low COMT activity increased capsaicin-induced pain perception in women, but not in men.	[167]

CONCLUSION

Multitudinous factors interact with each other for sensing the initial noxious signal, interpreting it and then collaborate with the natural internal analgesia of the body to announce the final verdict of pain. All this complex combinations within the brain engage physical, physiological and psychological triggers, but growing body of evidence suggests that sensory input is first and foremost realized, processed and mediated through an individual's genetic profile. Moreover, even the endogenous effect and efficacy of anti-nociceptive drugs depends upon the genes one carries. In the clinical chapters, decoding and interpreting the genetic signatures of pain in several pain conditions have heralded the idea that personalized medicine, where every individual can be treated according to the genetic endowment is not a distant dream.

CONFLICT OF INTEREST

The authors confirm that they have no conflict of interest to declare for this publication.

ACKNOWLEDGEMENTS

We are thankful to UGC-BSR fellowship awarded to Ms. Harjot Dhillon and UGC Major Research Project sanctioned to Dr. Puneetpal Singh.

REFERENCES

[1] Basbaum AI, Bautista DM, Scherrer G, Julius D. Cellular and molecular mechanisms of pain. Cell 2009; 139(2): 267-84.
[http://dx.doi.org/10.1016/j.cell.2009.09.028] [PMID: 19837031]

[2] Caterina MJ, Schumacher MA, Tominaga M, Rosen TA, Levine JD, Julius D. The capsaicin receptor: a heat-activated ion channel in the pain pathway. Nature 1997; 389(6653): 816-24.
[http://dx.doi.org/10.1038/39807] [PMID: 9349813]

[3] Tóth DM, Szoke E, Bölcskei K, *et al.* Nociception, neurogenic inflammation and thermoregulation in TRPV1 knockdown transgenic mice. Cell Mol Life Sci 2011; 68(15): 2589-601.
[http://dx.doi.org/10.1007/s00018-010-0569-2] [PMID: 21069423]

[4] Armero P, Muriel C, López M, Santos J, González-Sarmiento R. Analysis of TRPV1 gene polymorphisms in Spanish patients with neuropathic pain. Med Clin (Barc) 2012; 139(1): 1-4.
[http://dx.doi.org/10.1016/j.medcli.2011.10.028] [PMID: 22401740]

[5] Li L, Hasan R, Zhang X. The basal thermal sensitivity of the TRPV1 ion channel is determined by PKCβII. J Neurosci 2014; 34(24): 8246-58.
[http://dx.doi.org/10.1523/JNEUROSCI.0278-14.2014] [PMID: 24920628]

[6] Riera CE, Huising MO, Follett P, *et al.* TRPV1 pain receptors regulate longevity and metabolism by neuropeptide signaling. Cell 2014; 157(5): 1023-36.

[http://dx.doi.org/10.1016/j.cell.2014.03.051] [PMID: 24855942]

[7] Binder A, May D, Baron R, *et al.* Transient receptor potential channel polymorphisms are associated with the somatosensory function in neuropathic pain patients. PLoS One 2011; 6(3): e17387. [http://dx.doi.org/10.1371/journal.pone.0017387] [PMID: 21468319]

[8] Ochodnický P, Michel MB, Butter JJ, Seth J, Panicker JN, Michel MC. Bradykinin modulates spontaneous nerve growth factor production and stretch-induced ATP release in human urothelium. Pharmacol Res 2013; 70(1): 147-54. [http://dx.doi.org/10.1016/j.phrs.2013.01.010] [PMID: 23376352]

[9] Murase S, Terazawa E, Queme F, *et al.* Bradykinin and nerve growth factor play pivotal roles in muscular mechanical hyperalgesia after exercise (delayed-onset muscle soreness). J Neurosci 2010; 30(10): 3752-61. [http://dx.doi.org/10.1523/JNEUROSCI.3803-09.2010] [PMID: 20220009]

[10] de Oliveira Fusaro MC, Pelegrini-da-Silva A, Araldi D, Parada CA, Tambeli CH. P2X3 and P2X2/3 receptors mediate mechanical hyperalgesia induced by bradykinin, but not by pro-inflammatory cytokines, PGE_2 or dopamine. Eur J Pharmacol 2010; 649(1-3): 177-82. [http://dx.doi.org/10.1016/j.ejphar.2010.09.037] [PMID: 20868656]

[11] Cho H, Oh U. Anoctamin 1 mediates thermal pain as a heat sensor. Curr Neuropharmacol 2013; 11(6): 641-51. [http://dx.doi.org/10.2174/1570159X113119990038] [PMID: 24396339]

[12] Liu B, Linley JE, Du X, *et al.* The acute nociceptive signals induced by bradykinin in rat sensory neurons are mediated by inhibition of M-type K+ channels and activation of Ca2+-activated Cl-channels. J Clin Invest 2010; 120(4): 1240-52. [http://dx.doi.org/10.1172/JCI41084] [PMID: 20335661]

[13] Carreño O, Corominas R, Fernández-Morales J, *et al.* SNP variants within the vanilloid TRPV1 and TRPV3 receptor genes are associated with migraine in the Spanish population. Am J Med Genet B Neuropsychiatr Genet 2012; 159B(1): 94-103. [http://dx.doi.org/10.1002/ajmg.b.32007] [PMID: 22162417]

[14] Todaka H, Taniguchi J, Satoh J, Mizuno A, Suzuki M. Warm temperature-sensitive transient receptor potential vanilloid 4 (TRPV4) plays an essential role in thermal hyperalgesia. J Biol Chem 2004; 279(34): 35133-8. [http://dx.doi.org/10.1074/jbc.M406260200] [PMID: 15187078]

[15] May D, Baastrup J, Nientit MR, *et al.* Differential expression and functionality of TRPA1 protein genetic variants in conditions of thermal stimulation. J Biol Chem 2012; 287(32): 27087-94. [http://dx.doi.org/10.1074/jbc.M112.341776] [PMID: 22665484]

[16] Schütz M, Oertel BG, Heimann D, *et al.* Consequences of a human TRPA1 genetic variant on the perception of nociceptive and olfactory stimuli. PLoS One 2014; 9(4): e95592. [http://dx.doi.org/10.1371/journal.pone.0095592] [PMID: 24752136]

[17] Kim H, Mittal DP, Iadarola MJ, Dionne RA. Genetic predictors for acute experimental cold and heat pain sensitivity in humans. J Med Genet 2006; 43(8): e40. [http://dx.doi.org/10.1136/jmg.2005.036079] [PMID: 16882734]

[18] Treister R, Pud D, Ebstein RP, Eisenberg E. Dopamine transporter genotype dependent effects of apomorphine on cold pain tolerance in healthy volunteers. PLoS One 2013; 8(5): e63808. [http://dx.doi.org/10.1371/journal.pone.0063808] [PMID: 23704939]

[19] Lippoldt EK, Elmes RR, McCoy DD, Knowlton WM, McKemy DD. Artemin, a glial cell line-derived neurotrophic factor family member, induces TRPM8-dependent cold pain. J Neurosci 2013; 33(30): 12543-52. [http://dx.doi.org/10.1523/JNEUROSCI.5765-12.2013] [PMID: 23884957]

[20] Ren AJ, Wang K, Zhang H, *et al.* ZBTB20 regulates nociception and pain sensation by modulating TRP channel expression in nociceptive sensory neurons. Nat Commun 2014; 5: 4984. [http://dx.doi.org/10.1038/ncomms5984] [PMID: 25369838]

[21] Reimann F, Cox JJ, Belfer I, *et al.* Pain perception is altered by a nucleotide polymorphism in SCN9A. Proc Natl Acad Sci USA 2010; 107(11): 5148-53. [http://dx.doi.org/10.1073/pnas.0913181107] [PMID: 20212137]

[22] Cregg R, Momin A, Rugiero F, Wood JN. Pain channelopathies Physiol. Wood JN, Zhao J 2010; 588 (Pt 11)(1): 1897-904.

[23] Sun X, Jin J, Zhang JG, *et al.* Expression of acid-sensing ion channels in nucleus pulposus cells of the human intervertebral disk is regulated by non-steroid anti-inflammatory drugs. Acta Biochim Biophys Sin (Shanghai) 2014; 46(9): 774-81. [http://dx.doi.org/10.1093/abbs/gmu067] [PMID: 25079679]

[24] Ikeuchi M, Kolker SJ, Sluka KA. Acid-sensing ion channel 3 expression in mouse knee joint afferents and effects of carrageenan-induced arthritis. J Pain 2009; 10(3): 336-42. [http://dx.doi.org/10.1016/j.jpain.2008.10.010] [PMID: 19185546]

[25] Rash LD. ASIC3: first the heartache, now a migraine! Headache 2013; 53(8): 1204-6. [http://dx.doi.org/10.1111/head.12170] [PMID: 24020955]

[26] Qiu F, Qiu CY, Cai H, *et al.* Oxytocin inhibits the activity of acid-sensing ion channels through the vasopressin, V1A receptor in primary sensory neurons. Br J Pharmacol 2014; 171(12): 3065-76. [http://dx.doi.org/10.1111/bph.12635] [PMID: 24641084]

[27] Krimon S, Araldi D, do Prado FC, Tambeli CH, Oliveira-Fusaro MC, Parada CA. P2X3 receptors induced inflammatory nociception modulated by TRPA1, 5-HT3 and 5-HT1A receptors. Pharmacol Biochem Behav 2013; 112: 49-55. [http://dx.doi.org/10.1016/j.pbb.2013.09.017] [PMID: 24120766]

[28] Ide S, Nishizawa D, Fukuda K, *et al.* Haplotypes of P2RX7 gene polymorphisms are associated with both cold pain sensitivity and analgesic effect of fentanyl. Mol Pain 2014; 10: 75. [http://dx.doi.org/10.1186/1744-8069-10-75] [PMID: 25472448]

[29] Vinuela-Fernandez I, Sun L, Jerina H, *et al.* The TRPM8 channel forms a complex with the 5-HT(1B) receptor and phospholipase D that amplifies its reversal of pain hypersensitivity. Neuropharmacology 2014; 79: 136-51. [http://dx.doi.org/10.1016/j.neuropharm.2013.11.006] [PMID: 24269608]

[30] Lindstedt F, Karshikoff B, Schalling M, *et al.* Serotonin-1A receptor polymorphism (rs6295) associated with thermal pain perception. PLoS One 2012; 7(8): e43221.

[http://dx.doi.org/10.1371/journal.pone.0043221] [PMID: 22952650]

[31] Ugawa S, Ueda T, Ishida Y, Nishigaki M, Shibata Y, Shimada S. Amiloride-blockable acid-sensing ion channels are leading acid sensors expressed in human nociceptors. J Clin Invest 2002; 110(8): 1185-90.
[http://dx.doi.org/10.1172/JCI0215709] [PMID: 12393854]

[32] Jones NG, Slater R, Cadiou H, McNaughton P, McMahon SB. Acid-induced pain and its modulation in humans. J Neurosci 2004; 24(48): 10974-9.
[http://dx.doi.org/10.1523/JNEUROSCI.2619-04.2004] [PMID: 15574747]

[33] Maes M, Libbrecht I, Van Hunsel F, *et al.* The immune-inflammatory pathophysiology of fibromyalgia: increased serum soluble gp130, the common signal transducer protein of various neurotrophic cytokines. Psychoneuroendocrinology 1999; 24(4): 371-83.
[http://dx.doi.org/10.1016/S0306-4530(98)00087-0] [PMID: 10341365]

[34] Valdes AM, De Wilde G, Doherty SA, *et al.* The Ile585Val TRPV1 variant is involved in risk of painful knee osteoarthritis. Ann Rheum Dis 2011; 70(9): 1556-61.
[http://dx.doi.org/10.1136/ard.2010.148122] [PMID: 21616913]

[35] Emery EC, Young GT, Berrocoso EM, Chen L, McNaughton PA. HCN2 ion channels play a central role in inflammatory and neuropathic pain. Science 2011; 333(6048): 1462-6.
[http://dx.doi.org/10.1126/science.1206243] [PMID: 21903816]

[36] Ritter DM, Zemel BM, Hala TJ, O'Leary ME, Lepore AC, Covarrubias M. Dysregulation of Kv3.4 channels in dorsal root ganglia following spinal cord injury. J Neurosci 2015; 35(3): 1260-73.
[http://dx.doi.org/10.1523/JNEUROSCI.1594-14.2015] [PMID: 25609640]

[37] Tsantoulas C, Zhu L, Shaifta Y, *et al.* Sensory neuron downregulation of the Kv9.1 potassium channel subunit mediates neuropathic pain following nerve injury. J Neurosci 2012; 32(48): 17502-13.
[http://dx.doi.org/10.1523/JNEUROSCI.3561-12.2012] [PMID: 23197740]

[38] Bruehl S, Denton JS, Lonergan D, *et al.* Associations between KCNJ6 (GIRK2) gene polymorphisms and pain-related phenotypes. Pain 2013; 154(12): 2853-9.
[http://dx.doi.org/10.1016/j.pain.2013.08.026] [PMID: 23994450]

[39] Nockemann D, Rouault M, Labuz D, *et al.* The K(+) channel GIRK2 is both necessary and sufficient for peripheral opioid-mediated analgesia. EMBO Mol Med 2013; 5(8): 1263-77.
[http://dx.doi.org/10.1002/emmm.201201980] [PMID: 23818182]

[40] Marker CL, Luján R, Loh HH, Wickman K. Spinal G-protein-gated potassium channels contribute in a dose-dependent manner to the analgesic effect of mu- and delta- but not kappa-opioids. J Neurosci 2005; 25(14): 3551-9.
[http://dx.doi.org/10.1523/JNEUROSCI.4899-04.2005] [PMID: 15814785]

[41] Ikeda K, Kobayashi T, Kumanishi T, Yano R, Sora I, Niki H. Molecular mechanisms of analgesia induced by opioids and ethanol: is the GIRK channel one of the keys? Neurosci Res 2002; 44(2): 121-31.
[http://dx.doi.org/10.1016/S0168-0102(02)00094-9] [PMID: 12354627]

[42] Kobayashi T, Ikeda K, Kojima H, *et al.* Ethanol opens G-protein-activated inwardly rectifying K+ channels. Nat Neurosci 1999; 2(12): 1091-7.

[http://dx.doi.org/10.1038/16019] [PMID: 10570486]

[43] Chung MK, Cho YS, Bae YC, Lee J, Zhang X, Ro JY. Peripheral G protein-coupled inwardly rectifying potassium channels are involved in δ-opioid receptor-mediated anti-hyperalgesia in rat masseter muscle. Eur J Pain 2014; 18(1): 29-38.
[http://dx.doi.org/10.1002/j.1532-2149.2013.00343.x] [PMID: 23740773]

[44] Lötsch J, Prüss H, Veh RW, Doehring A. A KCNJ6 (Kir3.2, GIRK2) gene polymorphism modulates opioid effects on analgesia and addiction but not on pupil size. Pharmacogenet Genomics 2010; 20(5): 291-7.
[http://dx.doi.org/10.1097/FPC.0b013e3283386bda] [PMID: 20220551]

[45] Nishizawa D, Nagashima M, Katoh R, *et al.* Association between KCNJ6 (GIRK2) gene polymorphisms and postoperative analgesic requirements after major abdominal surgery. PLoS One 2009; 4(9): e7060.
[http://dx.doi.org/10.1371/journal.pone.0007060] [PMID: 19756153]

[46] Chiou LC, Liao YY, Guerrini R, Calo' G. [Nphe1,Arg14,Lys15]N/OFQ-NH2 is a competitive antagonist of NOP receptors in the periaqueductal gray. Eur J Pharmacol 2005; 515(1-3): 47-53.
[http://dx.doi.org/10.1016/j.ejphar.2005.03.036] [PMID: 15896734]

[47] Wang W, Atianjoh F, Gauda EB, Yaster M, Li Y, Tao YX. Increased expression of sodium channel subunit Nav1.1 in the injured dorsal root ganglion after peripheral nerve injury. Anat Rec (Hoboken) 2011; 294(8): 1406-11.
[http://dx.doi.org/10.1002/ar.21437] [PMID: 21714116]

[48] Fryatt AG, Mulheran M, Egerton J, Gunthorpe MJ, Grubb BD. Ototrauma induces sodium channel plasticity in auditory afferent neurons. Mol Cell Neurosci 2011; 48(1): 51-61.
[http://dx.doi.org/10.1016/j.mcn.2011.06.005] [PMID: 21708262]

[49] Alvarado S, Tajerian M, Millecamps M, Suderman M, Stone LS, Szyf M. Peripheral nerve injury is accompanied by chronic transcriptome-wide changes in the mouse prefrontal cortex. Mol Pain 2013; 9: 21.
[http://dx.doi.org/10.1186/1744-8069-9-21] [PMID: 23597049]

[50] Deuis JR, Zimmermann K, Romanovsky AA, *et al.* An animal model of oxaliplatin-induced cold allodynia reveals a crucial role for Nav1.6 in peripheral pain pathways. Pain 2013; 154(9): 1749-57.
[http://dx.doi.org/10.1016/j.pain.2013.05.032] [PMID: 23711479]

[51] Shirahata E, Iwasaki H, Takagi M, *et al.* Ankyrin-G regulates inactivation gating of the neuronal sodium channel, Nav1.6. J Neurophysiol 2006; 96(3): 1347-57.
[http://dx.doi.org/10.1152/jn.01264.2005] [PMID: 16775201]

[52] Jarecki BW, Piekarz AD, Jackson JO II, Cummins TR. Human voltage-gated sodium channel mutations that cause inherited neuronal and muscle channelopathies increase resurgent sodium currents. J Clin Invest 2010; 120(1): 369-78.
[http://dx.doi.org/10.1172/JCI40801] [PMID: 20038812]

[53] Hoeijmakers JG, Faber CG, Merkies IS, Waxman SG. Painful peripheral neuropathy and sodium channel mutations. Neurosci Lett 2015; 596: 51-9.
[http://dx.doi.org/10.1016/j.neulet.2014.12.056] [PMID: 25556685]

[54] Gudes S, Barkai O, Caspi Y, Katz B, Lev S, Binshtok AM. The role of slow and persistent TTX-resistant sodium currents in acute tumor necrosis factor-α-mediated increase in nociceptors excitability. J Neurophysiol 2015; 113(2): 601-19.
[http://dx.doi.org/10.1152/jn.00652.2014] [PMID: 25355965]

[55] Christidis N, Kang I, Cairns BE, *et al.* Expression of 5-HT3 receptors and TTX resistant sodium channels (Na(V)1.8) on muscle nerve fibers in pain-free humans and patients with chronic myofascial temporomandibular disorders. J Headache Pain 2014; 15: 63.
[http://dx.doi.org/10.1186/1129-2377-15-63] [PMID: 25261281]

[56] Huang J, Yang Y, Dib-Hajj SD, *et al.* Depolarized inactivation overcomes impaired activation to produce DRG neuron hyperexcitability in a Nav1.7 mutation in a patient with distal limb pain. J Neurosci 2014; 34(37): 12328-40.
[http://dx.doi.org/10.1523/JNEUROSCI.2773-14.2014] [PMID: 25209274]

[57] Mo G, Grant R, O'Donnell D, Ragsdale DS, Cao CQ, Séguéla P. Neuropathic Nav1.3-mediated sensitization to P2X activation is regulated by protein kinase C. Mol Pain 2011; 7: 14.
[http://dx.doi.org/10.1186/1744-8069-7-14] [PMID: 21314936]

[58] Ding Y, Cesare P, Drew L, Nikitaki D, Wood JN. ATP, P2X receptors and pain pathways. J Auton Nerv Syst 2000; 81(1-3): 289-94.
[http://dx.doi.org/10.1016/S0165-1838(00)00131-4] [PMID: 10869734]

[59] Liu S, Shi Q, Zhu Q, *et al.* $P2X_7$ receptor of rat dorsal root ganglia is involved in the effect of moxibustion on visceral hyperalgesia. Purinergic Signal 2015; 11(2): 161-9.
[http://dx.doi.org/10.1007/s11302-014-9439-y] [PMID: 25527178]

[60] Schuelert N, Just S, Corradini L, Kuelzer R, Bernloehr C, Doods H. The bradykinin B1 receptor antagonist BI113823 reverses inflammatory hyperalgesia by desensitization of peripheral and spinal neurons. Eur J Pain 2015; 19(1): 132-42.
[http://dx.doi.org/10.1002/ejp.573] [PMID: 25088373]

[61] Lee B, Cho H, Jung J, Yang YD, Yang DJ, Oh U. Anoctamin 1 contributes to inflammatory and nerve-injury induced hypersensitivity. Mol Pain 2014; 10: 5.
[http://dx.doi.org/10.1186/1744-8069-10-5] [PMID: 24450308]

[62] Schistad EI, Jacobsen LM, Røe C, Gjerstad J. The interleukin-1α gene C>T polymorphism rs1800587 is associated with increased pain intensity and decreased pressure pain thresholds in patients with lumbar radicular pain. Clin J Pain 2014; 30(10): 869-74.
[http://dx.doi.org/10.1097/AJP.0000000000000048] [PMID: 24300227]

[63] Leipe J, Schramm MA, Prots I, Schulze-Koops H, Skapenko A. Increased Th17 cell frequency and poor clinical outcome in rheumatoid arthritis are associated with a genetic variant in the IL4R gene, rs1805010. Arthritis Rheumatol 2014; 66(5): 1165-75.
[http://dx.doi.org/10.1002/art.38343] [PMID: 24782180]

[64] Shi LP, He Y, Liu ZD. Correlation between single nucleotide polymorphism of rs3811047 in IL-1 F7 gene and rheumatoid arthritis susceptibility among Han population in central plains of China. Asian Pac J Trop Med 2013; 6(1): 73-5.
[http://dx.doi.org/10.1016/S1995-7645(12)60204-1] [PMID: 23317890]

[65] Pei B, Xu S, Liu T, Pan F, Xu J, Ding C. Associations of the IL-1F7 gene polymorphisms with rheumatoid arthritis in Chinese Han population. Int J Immunogenet 2013; 40(3): 199-203. [http://dx.doi.org/10.1111/iji.12007] [PMID: 23171316]

[66] Benemei S, Nicoletti P, Capone JG, Geppetti P. CGRP receptors in the control of pain and inflammation. Curr Opin Pharmacol 2009; 9(1): 9-14. [http://dx.doi.org/10.1016/j.coph.2008.12.007] [PMID: 19157980]

[67] Salio C, Ferrini F, Muthuraju S, Merighi A. Presynaptic modulation of spinal nociceptive transmission by glial cell line-derived neurotrophic factor (GDNF). J Neurosci 2014; 34(41): 13819-33. [http://dx.doi.org/10.1523/JNEUROSCI.0808-14.2014] [PMID: 25297108]

[68] Kohli U, Muszkat M, Sofowora GG, *et al.* Effects of variation in the human alpha2A- and alpha2C-adrenoceptor genes on cognitive tasks and pain perception. Eur J Pain 2010; 14(2): 154-9. [http://dx.doi.org/10.1016/j.ejpain.2009.04.003] [PMID: 19423370]

[69] Ahmed AZ, El-Shahaly HA, Omar AS, Ghattas MH. Patterns of angiotensin converting enzyme insertion/deletion gene polymorphism among an Egyptian cohort of patients with rheumatoid arthritis. Int J Rheum Dis 2013; 16(3): 284-90. [http://dx.doi.org/10.1111/j.1756-185X.2012.01820.x] [PMID: 23981749]

[70] Inanır A, Yigit S, Tural S, Ozturk SD, Akkanet S, Habiboğlu A. Significant association between insertion/deletion polymorphism of the angiotensin-convertig enzyme gene and ankylosing spondylitis. Mol Vis 2012; 18: 2107-13. [PMID: 22876137]

[71] Inanir A, Yigit S, Tural S, Cecen O, Yildirim E. MTHFR gene C677T mutation and ACE gene I/D polymorphism in Turkish patients with osteoarthritis. Dis Markers 2013; 34(1): 17-22. [http://dx.doi.org/10.1155/2013/658654] [PMID: 23089924]

[72] Solovieva S, Leino-Arjas P, Saarela J, Luoma K, Raininko R, Riihimäki H. Possible association of interleukin 1 gene locus polymorphisms with low back pain. Pain 2004; 109(1-2): 8-19. [http://dx.doi.org/10.1016/j.pain.2003.10.020] [PMID: 15082121]

[73] Paz Aparicio J, Fernández Bances I, López-Anglada Fernández E, *et al.* The IL-1β (+3953 T/C) gene polymorphism associates to symptomatic lumbar disc herniation. Eur Spine J 2011; 20 (Suppl. 3): 383-9. [http://dx.doi.org/10.1007/s00586-011-1915-2] [PMID: 21837414]

[74] Oen K, Malleson PN, Cabral DA, *et al.* Cytokine genotypes correlate with pain and radiologically defined joint damage in patients with juvenile rheumatoid arthritis. Rheumatology (Oxford) 2005; 44(9): 1115-21. [http://dx.doi.org/10.1093/rheumatology/keh689] [PMID: 15901906]

[75] Shi LP, He Y, Liu ZD. Correlation between single nucleotide polymorphism of rs3811047 in IL-1 F7 gene and rheumatoid arthritis susceptibility among Han population in central plains of China. Asian Pac J Trop Med 2013; 6(1): 73-5. [http://dx.doi.org/10.1016/S1995-7645(12)60204-1] [PMID: 23317890]

[76] Matute Wilander A, Kåredal M, Axmon A, Nordander C. Inflammatory biomarkers in serum in subjects with and without work related neck/shoulder complaints. BMC Musculoskelet Disord 2014;

15: 103.
[http://dx.doi.org/10.1186/1471-2474-15-103] [PMID: 24669872]

[77] Feng J, Zhang Z, Wu X, *et al.* Discovery of potential new gene variants and inflammatory cytokine associations with fibromyalgia syndrome by whole exome sequencing. PLoS One 2013; 8(6): e65033. [http://dx.doi.org/10.1371/journal.pone.0065033] [PMID: 23762283]

[78] Arendt-Nielsen L, Eskehave TN, Egsgaard LL, *et al.* Association between experimental pain biomarkers and serologic markers in patients with different degrees of painful knee osteoarthritis. Arthritis Rheumatol 2014; 66(12): 3317-26.
[http://dx.doi.org/10.1002/art.38856] [PMID: 25168637]

[79] Peciña M, Martínez-Jauand M, Love T, *et al.* Valence-specific effects of BDNF Val66Met polymorphism on dopaminergic stress and reward processing in humans. J Neurosci 2014; 34(17): 5874-81.
[http://dx.doi.org/10.1523/JNEUROSCI.2152-13.2014] [PMID: 24760847]

[80] Xiao Y, Russell IJ, Liu YG. A brain-derived neurotrophic factor polymorphism Val66Met identifies fibromyalgia syndrome subgroup with higher body mass index and C-reactive protein. Rheumatol Int 2012; 32(8): 2479-85.
[http://dx.doi.org/10.1007/s00296-011-1990-z] [PMID: 21773883]

[81] Haas L, Portela LV, Böhmer AE, Oses JP, Lara DR. Increased plasma levels of brain derived neurotrophic factor (BDNF) in patients with fibromyalgia. Neurochem Res 2010; 35(5): 830-4. [http://dx.doi.org/10.1007/s11064-010-0129-z] [PMID: 20119637]

[82] Reimann F, Cox JJ, Belfer I, *et al.* Pain perception is altered by a nucleotide polymorphism in SCN9A. Proc Natl Acad Sci USA 2010; 107(11): 5148-53.
[http://dx.doi.org/10.1073/pnas.0913181107] [PMID: 20212137]

[83] Duan G, Xiang G, Zhang X, Yuan R, Zhan H, Qi D. A single-nucleotide polymorphism in SCN9A may decrease postoperative pain sensitivity in the general population. Anesthesiology 2013; 118(2): 436-42.
[http://dx.doi.org/10.1097/ALN.0b013e31827dde74] [PMID: 23364568]

[84] Heimann D, Lötsch J, Hummel T, Doehring A, Oertel BG. Linkage between increased nociception and olfaction *via* a SCN9A haplotype. PLoS One 2013; 8(7): e68654.
[http://dx.doi.org/10.1371/journal.pone.0068654] [PMID: 23874707]

[85] Zhang XY, Wen J, Yang W, *et al.* Gain-of-function mutations in SCN11A cause familial episodic pain. Am J Hum Genet 2013; 93(5): 957-66.
[http://dx.doi.org/10.1016/j.ajhg.2013.09.016] [PMID: 24207120]

[86] Costigan M, Belfer I, Griffin RS, *et al.* Multiple chronic pain states are associated with a common amino acid-changing allele in KCNS1. Brain 2010; 133(9): 2519-27.
[http://dx.doi.org/10.1093/brain/awq195] [PMID: 20724292]

[87] Bruehl S, Denton JS, Lonergan D, *et al.* Associations between KCNJ6 (GIRK2) gene polymorphisms and pain-related phenotypes. Pain 2013; 154(12): 2853-9.
[http://dx.doi.org/10.1016/j.pain.2013.08.026] [PMID: 23994450]

[88] Rukwied R, Chizh BA, Lorenz U, *et al.* Potentiation of nociceptive responses to low pH injections in

humans by prostaglandin E2. J Pain 2007; 8(5): 443-51.
[http://dx.doi.org/10.1016/j.jpain.2006.12.004] [PMID: 17337250]

[89] Omair A, Holden M, Lie BA, Reikeras O, Brox JI. Treatment outcome of chronic low back pain and radiographic lumbar disc degeneration are associated with inflammatory and matrix degrading gene variants: a prospective genetic association study. BMC Musculoskelet Disord 2013; 14: 105.
[http://dx.doi.org/10.1186/1471-2474-14-105] [PMID: 23522322]

[90] Noponen-Hietala N, Virtanen I, Karttunen R, *et al.* Genetic variations in IL6 associate with intervertebral disc disease characterized by sciatica. Pain 2005; 114(1-2): 186-94.
[http://dx.doi.org/10.1016/j.pain.2004.12.015] [PMID: 15733644]

[91] İnal EE, Görükmez O, Eroğlu S, *et al.* Association of GSTM1, GSTT1, GSTP1-ILE105VAL and ACE I/D polymorphisms with ankylosing spondylitis Rheumatol Int 2015. Ahead of print

[92] Chung OY, Bruehl S, Diedrich L, Diedrich A, Chont M, Robertson D. Baroreflex sensitivity associated hypoalgesia in healthy states is altered by chronic pain. Pain 2008; 138(1): 87-97.
[http://dx.doi.org/10.1016/j.pain.2007.11.011] [PMID: 18164819]

[93] Campbell CM, Edwards RR, Carmona C, *et al.* Polymorphisms in the GTP cyclohydrolase gene (GCH1) are associated with ratings of capsaicin pain. Pain 2009; 141(1-2): 114-8.
[http://dx.doi.org/10.1016/j.pain.2008.10.023] [PMID: 19081190]

[94] Schizas N, Lian Ø, Frihagen F, Engebretsen L, Bahr R, Ackermann PW. Coexistence of up-regulated NMDA receptor 1 and glutamate on nerves, vessels and transformed tenocytes in tendinopathy. Scand J Med Sci Sports 2010; 20(2): 208-15.
[http://dx.doi.org/10.1111/j.1600-0838.2009.00913.x] [PMID: 19422642]

[95] Schizas N, Weiss R, Lian O, Frihagen F, Bahr R, Ackermann PW. Glutamate receptors in tendinopathic patients. J Orthop Res 2012; 30(9): 1447-52.
[http://dx.doi.org/10.1002/jor.22094] [PMID: 22354721]

[96] Hood DD, Mallak KA, James RL, Tuttle R, Eisenach JC. Enhancement of analgesia from systemic opioid in humans by spinal cholinesterase inhibition. J Pharmacol Exp Ther 1997; 282(1): 86-92.
[PMID: 9223543]

[97] Danielson P, Andersson G, Alfredson H, Forsgren S. Extensive expression of markers for acetylcholine synthesis and of M2 receptors in tenocytes in therapy-resistant chronic painful patellar tendon tendinosis - a pilot study. Life Sci 2007; 80(24-25): 2235-8.
[http://dx.doi.org/10.1016/j.lfs.2007.01.005] [PMID: 17289083]

[98] Rhodin A, Grönbladh A, Ginya H, *et al.* Combined analysis of circulating β-endorphin with gene polymorphisms in OPRM1, CACNAD2 and ABCB1 reveals correlation with pain, opioid sensitivity and opioid-related side effects. Mol Brain 2013; 6: 8.
[http://dx.doi.org/10.1186/1756-6606-6-8] [PMID: 23402298]

[99] Taylor CP. Mechanisms of analgesia by gabapentin and pregabalin--calcium channel alpha2-delta [Cavalpha2-delta] ligands. Pain 2009; 142(1-2): 13-6.
[http://dx.doi.org/10.1016/j.pain.2008.11.019] [PMID: 19128880]

[100] Treister R, Pud D, Ebstein RP, *et al.* Associations between polymorphisms in dopamine neurotransmitter pathway genes and pain response in healthy humans. Pain 2009; 147(1-3): 187-93.

[http://dx.doi.org/10.1016/j.pain.2009.09.001] [PMID: 19796878]

[101] Almanza A, Simón-Arceo K, Coffeen U, *et al.* A D2-like receptor family agonist produces analgesia in mechanonociception but not in thermonociception at the spinal cord level in rats. Pharmacol Biochem Behav 2015; 137: 119-25.
[http://dx.doi.org/10.1016/j.pbb.2015.08.013] [PMID: 26303304]

[102] Wood PB, Schweinhardt P, Jaeger E, *et al.* Fibromyalgia patients show an abnormal dopamine response to pain. Eur J Neurosci 2007; 25(12): 3576-82.
[http://dx.doi.org/10.1111/j.1460-9568.2007.05623.x] [PMID: 17610577]

[103] Zhuo M, Gebhart GF. Spinal serotonin receptors mediate descending facilitation of a nociceptive reflex from the nuclei reticularis gigantocellularis and gigantocellularis pars alpha in the rat. Brain Res 1991; 550(1): 35-48.
[http://dx.doi.org/10.1016/0006-8993(91)90402-H] [PMID: 1888999]

[104] Miller LE, Grifka J, Schölmerich J, Straub RH. Norepinephrine from synovial tyrosine hydroxylase positive cells is a strong indicator of synovial inflammation in rheumatoid arthritis. J Rheumatol 2002; 29(3): 427-35. [Erratum in: J Rheumatol 2003; 30:1125].
[PMID: 11908553]

[105] Miller LE, Jüsten HP, Schölmerich J, Straub RH. The loss of sympathetic nerve fibers in the synovial tissue of patients with rheumatoid arthritis is accompanied by increased norepinephrine release from synovial macrophages. FASEB J 2000; 14(13): 2097-107.
[http://dx.doi.org/10.1096/fj.99-1082com] [PMID: 11023994]

[106] Oehmke MJ, Podranski T, Mann M, Frickey N, Kuhn DF, Hempelmann G. Perioperative concentrations of catecholamines in the cerebrospinal fluid and plasma during spinal anesthesia. Acta Anaesthesiol Scand 2008; 52(4): 487-92.
[http://dx.doi.org/10.1111/j.1399-6576.2007.01551.x] [PMID: 18339154]

[107] Quax RA, de Man YA, Koper JW, *et al.* Glucocorticoid receptor gene polymorphisms and disease activity during pregnancy and the postpartum period in rheumatoid arthritis. Arthritis Res Ther 2012; 14(4): R183.
[http://dx.doi.org/10.1186/ar4014] [PMID: 22889053]

[108] Quax RA, Koper JW, de Jong PH, *et al. In vitro* glucocorticoid sensitivity is associated with clinical glucocorticoid therapy outcome in rheumatoid arthritis. Arthritis Res Ther 2012; 14(4): R195.
[http://dx.doi.org/10.1186/ar4029] [PMID: 22920577]

[109] Liu ZL, Ma H, Xu RX, *et al.* Potassium channels underlie postsynaptic but not presynaptic GABAB receptor-mediated inhibition on ventrolateral periaqueductal gray neurons. Brain Res Bull 2012; 88(5): 529-33.
[http://dx.doi.org/10.1016/j.brainresbull.2012.05.010] [PMID: 22634546]

[110] Huang CJ, Liu HF, Su NY, *et al.* Association between human opioid receptor genes polymorphisms and pressure pain sensitivity in females. Anaesthesia 2008; 63(12): 1288-95.
[http://dx.doi.org/10.1111/j.1365-2044.2008.05760.x] [PMID: 19032295]

[111] Fillingim RB, Kaplan L, Staud R, *et al.* The A118G single nucleotide polymorphism of the mu-opioid receptor gene (OPRM1) is associated with pressure pain sensitivity in humans. J Pain 2005; 6(3): 159-67.

[http://dx.doi.org/10.1016/j.jpain.2004.11.008] [PMID: 15772909]

[112] Chou WY, Yang LC, Lu HF, *et al.* Association of mu-opioid receptor gene polymorphism (A118G) with variations in morphine consumption for analgesia after total knee arthroplasty. Acta Anaesthesiol Scand 2006; 50(7): 787-92.
[http://dx.doi.org/10.1111/j.1399-6576.2006.01058.x] [PMID: 16879459]

[113] Mishra BK, Wu T, Belfer I, *et al.* Do motor control genes contribute to interindividual variability in decreased movement in patients with pain? Mol Pain 2007; 3: 20.
[http://dx.doi.org/10.1186/1744-8069-3-20] [PMID: 17655760]

[114] Fillingim RB, Kaplan L, Staud R, *et al.* The A118G single nucleotide polymorphism of the mu-opioid receptor gene (OPRM1) is associated with pressure pain sensitivity in humans. J Pain 2005; 6(3): 159-67.
[http://dx.doi.org/10.1016/j.jpain.2004.11.008] [PMID: 15772909]

[115] Chou WY, Yang LC, Lu HF, *et al.* Association of mu-opioid receptor gene polymorphism (A118G) with variations in morphine consumption for analgesia after total knee arthroplasty. Acta Anaesthesiol Scand 2006; 50(7): 787-92.
[http://dx.doi.org/10.1111/j.1399-6576.2006.01058.x] [PMID: 16879459]

[116] Zwisler ST, Enggaard TP, Noehr-Jensen L, *et al.* The antinociceptive effect and adverse drug reactions of oxycodone in human experimental pain in relation to genetic variations in the OPRM1 and ABCB1 genes. Fundam Clin Pharmacol 2010; 24(4): 517-24.
[http://dx.doi.org/10.1111/j.1472-8206.2009.00781.x] [PMID: 19845769]

[117] Molliver DC, Rau KK, McIlwrath SL, Jankowski MP, Koerber HR. The ADP receptor P2Y1 is necessary for normal thermal sensitivity in cutaneous polymodal nociceptors. Mol Pain 2011; 7: 13.
[http://dx.doi.org/10.1186/1744-8069-7-13] [PMID: 21310055]

[118] Horváth G, Gölöncsér F, Csölle C, *et al.* Central P2Y12 receptor blockade alleviates inflammatory and neuropathic pain and cytokine production in rodents. Neurobiol Dis 2014; 70: 162-78.
[http://dx.doi.org/10.1016/j.nbd.2014.06.011] [PMID: 24971933]

[119] Tsuda M, Tozaki-Saitoh H, Inoue K. Purinergic system, microglia and neuropathic pain. Curr Opin Pharmacol 2012; 12(1): 74-9.
[http://dx.doi.org/10.1016/j.coph.2011.10.014] [PMID: 22036170]

[120] Taylor BK, Fu W, Kuphal KE, *et al.* Inflammation enhances Y1 receptor signaling, neuropeptide Y-mediated inhibition of hyperalgesia, and substance P release from primary afferent neurons. Neuroscience 2014; 256: 178-94.
[http://dx.doi.org/10.1016/j.neuroscience.2013.10.054] [PMID: 24184981]

[121] Lee YS, Kim H, Wu TX, Wang XM, Dionne RA. Genetically mediated interindividual variation in analgesic responses to cyclooxygenase inhibitory drugs. Clin Pharmacol Ther 2006; 79(5): 407-18.
[http://dx.doi.org/10.1016/j.clpt.2006.01.013] [PMID: 16678543]

[122] Meotti FC, Campos R, da Silva K, Paszcuk AF, Costa R, Calixto JB. Inflammatory muscle pain is dependent on the activation of kinin B_1 and B_2 receptors and intracellular kinase pathways. Br J Pharmacol 2012; 166(3): 1127-39.
[http://dx.doi.org/10.1111/j.1476-5381.2012.01830.x] [PMID: 22220695]

[123] Anghel A, Taranu G, Seclaman E, *et al.* Safety of vascular endothelial and hepatocyte growth factor gene therapy in patients with critical limb ischemia. Curr Neurovasc Res 2011; 8(3): 183-9. [http://dx.doi.org/10.2174/156720211796558050] [PMID: 21675956]

[124] Seidel MF, Fiebich BL, Ulrich-Merzenich G, Candelario-Jalil E, Koch FW, Vetter H. Serotonin mediates PGE2 overexpression through 5-HT2A and 5-HT3 receptor subtypes in serum-free tissue culture of macrophage-like synovial cells. Rheumatol Int 2008; 28(10): 1017-22. [http://dx.doi.org/10.1007/s00296-008-0564-1] [PMID: 18368410]

[125] Tambeli CH, Oliveira MC, Clemente JT, Pelegrini-da-Silva A, Parada CA. A novel mechanism involved in 5-hydroxytryptamine-induced nociception: the indirect activation of primary afferents. Neuroscience 2006; 141(3): 1517-24. [http://dx.doi.org/10.1016/j.neuroscience.2006.04.030] [PMID: 16750893]

[126] Treister R, Pud D, Ebstein RP, *et al.* Association between polymorphisms in serotonin and dopamine-related genes and endogenous pain modulation. J Pain 2011; 12(8): 875-83. [http://dx.doi.org/10.1016/j.jpain.2011.02.348] [PMID: 21719351]

[127] Neziri AY, Dickenmann M, Scaramozzino P, *et al.* Effect of intravenous tropisetron on modulation of pain and central hypersensitivity in chronic low back pain patients. Pain 2012; 153(2): 311-8. [http://dx.doi.org/10.1016/j.pain.2011.10.008] [PMID: 22100357]

[128] Horjales-Araujo E, Demontis D, Lund EK, *et al.* Polymorphism in serotonin receptor 3B is associated with pain catastrophizing. PLoS One 2013; 8(11): e78889. [http://dx.doi.org/10.1371/journal.pone.0078889] [PMID: 24244382]

[129] Nicholl BI, Holliday KL, Macfarlane GJ, *et al.* Association of HTR2A polymorphisms with chronic widespread pain and the extent of musculoskeletal pain: results from two population-based cohorts. Arthritis Rheum 2011; 63(3): 810-8. [http://dx.doi.org/10.1002/art.30185] [PMID: 21305503]

[130] Oliveira MC, Pelegrini-da-Silva A, Parada CA, Tambeli CH. 5-HT acts on nociceptive primary afferents through an indirect mechanism to induce hyperalgesia in the subcutaneous tissue. Neuroscience 2007; 145(2): 708-14. [http://dx.doi.org/10.1016/j.neuroscience.2006.12.021] [PMID: 17257768]

[131] Bao L, Jin SX, Zhang C, *et al.* Activation of delta opioid receptors induces receptor insertion and neuropeptide secretion. Neuron 2003; 37(1): 121-33. [http://dx.doi.org/10.1016/S0896-6273(02)01103-0] [PMID: 12526778]

[132] Yin YW, Sun QQ, Hu AM, Wang Q, Liu HL. Association of rs9340799 polymorphism in estrogen receptor alpha gene with the risk of osteoarthritis: evidence based on 8,792 subjects. Mol Genet Genomics 2015; 290(2): 513-20. [http://dx.doi.org/10.1007/s00438-014-0940-3] [PMID: 25325995]

[133] Rut M, Machoy-Mokrzyńska A, Ręcławowicz D, *et al.* Influence of variation in the catechol--methyltransferase gene on the clinical outcome after lumbar spine surgery for one-level symptomatic disc disease: a report on 176 cases. Acta Neurochir (Wien) 2014; 156(2): 245-52. [http://dx.doi.org/10.1007/s00701-013-1895-6] [PMID: 24178190]

[134] Gupta R, Kumar V, Luthra K, Banerjee B, Bhatia MS. Polymorphism in apolipoprotein E among

migraineurs and tension-type headache subjects. J Headache Pain 2009; 10(2): 115-20. [http://dx.doi.org/10.1007/s10194-008-0094-y] [PMID: 19184578]

[135] Reeser JC, Payne E, Kitchner T, McCarty CA. Apolipoprotein e4 genotype increases the risk of being diagnosed with posttraumatic fibromyalgia. PM R 2011; 3(3): 193-7. [http://dx.doi.org/10.1016/j.pmrj.2010.12.009] [PMID: 21402364]

[136] Becker RM, da Silva VK, Machado FdaS, *et al.* Association between environmental quality, stress and APOE gene variation in fibromyalgia susceptibility determination. Rev Bras Reumatol 2010; 50(6): 617-24. [http://dx.doi.org/10.1590/S0482-50042010000600003] [PMID: 21243303]

[137] Lötsch J, von Hentig N, Freynhagen R, *et al.* Cross-sectional analysis of the influence of currently known pharmacogenetic modulators on opioid therapy in outpatient pain centers. Pharmacogenet Genomics 2009; 19(6): 429-36. [http://dx.doi.org/10.1097/FPC.0b013e32832b89da] [PMID: 19514130]

[138] Samer CF, Daali Y, Wagner M, *et al.* Genetic polymorphisms and drug interactions modulating CYP2D6 and CYP3A activities have a major effect on oxycodone analgesic efficacy and safety. Br J Pharmacol 2010; 160(4): 919-30. [http://dx.doi.org/10.1111/j.1476-5381.2010.00709.x] [PMID: 20590588]

[139] Peciña M, Martínez-Jauand M, Hodgkinson C, Stohler CS, Goldman D, Zubieta JK. FAAH selectively influences placebo effects. Mol Psychiatry 2014; 19(3): 385-91. [http://dx.doi.org/10.1038/mp.2013.124] [PMID: 24042479]

[140] Lindstedt F, Lonsdorf TB, Schalling M, Kosek E, Ingvar M. Perception of thermal pain and the thermal grill illusion is associated with polymorphisms in the serotonin transporter gene. PLoS One 2011; 6(3): e17752. [http://dx.doi.org/10.1371/journal.pone.0017752] [PMID: 21423614]

[141] Tegeder I, Adolph J, Schmidt H, Woolf CJ, Geisslinger G, Lötsch J. Reduced hyperalgesia in homozygous carriers of a GTP cyclohydrolase 1 haplotype. Eur J Pain 2008; 12(8): 1069-77. [http://dx.doi.org/10.1016/j.ejpain.2008.02.004] [PMID: 18374612]

[142] Holliday KL, Nicholl BI, Macfarlane GJ, Thomson W, Davies KA, McBeth J. Genetic variation in the hypothalamic-pituitary-adrenal stress axis influences susceptibility to musculoskeletal pain: results from the EPIFUND study. Ann Rheum Dis 2010; 69(3): 556-60. [http://dx.doi.org/10.1136/ard.2009.116137] [PMID: 19723618]

[143] Holliday KL, Nicholl BI, Macfarlane GJ, Thomson W, Davies KA, McBeth J. Do genetic predictors of pain sensitivity associate with persistent widespread pain? Mol Pain 2009; 5: 56. [http://dx.doi.org/10.1186/1744-8069-5-56] [PMID: 19775452]

[144] Potvin S, Larouche A, Normand E, *et al.* DRD3 Ser9Gly polymorphism is related to thermal pain perception and modulation in chronic widespread pain patients and healthy controls. J Pain 2009; 10(9): 969-75. [http://dx.doi.org/10.1016/j.jpain.2009.03.013] [PMID: 19464960]

[145] Ho AM, Tang NL, Cheung BK, Stadlin A. Dopamine receptor D4 gene -521C/T polymorphism is associated with opioid dependence through cold-pain responses. Ann N Y Acad Sci 2008; 1139: 20-6. [http://dx.doi.org/10.1196/annals.1432.054] [PMID: 18991844]

[146] Cargnin S, Magnani F, Viana M, *et al.* An opposite-direction modulation of the COMT Val158Met polymorphism on the clinical response to intrathecal morphine and triptans. J Pain 2013; 14(10): 1097-106.
[http://dx.doi.org/10.1016/j.jpain.2013.04.006] [PMID: 23773341]

[147] Desmeules J, Chabert J, Rebsamen M, *et al.* Central pain sensitization, COMT Val158Met polymorphism, and emotional factors in fibromyalgia. J Pain 2014; 15(2): 129-35.
[http://dx.doi.org/10.1016/j.jpain.2013.10.004] [PMID: 24342707]

[148] Fernández-de-Las-Peñas C, Ambite-Quesada S, Gil-Crujera A, Cigarán-Méndez M, Peñacoba-Puente C. Catechol-O-methyltransferase Val158Met polymorphism influences anxiety, depression, and disability, but not pressure pain sensitivity, in women with fibromyalgia syndrome. J Pain 2012; 13(11): 1068-74.
[http://dx.doi.org/10.1016/j.jpain.2012.08.001] [PMID: 23025981]

[149] Omair A, Lie BA, Reikeras O, Holden M, Brox JI. Genetic contribution of catechol--methyltransferase variants in treatment outcome of low back pain: a prospective genetic association study. BMC Musculoskelet Disord 2012; 13: 76.
[http://dx.doi.org/10.1186/1471-2474-13-76] [PMID: 22612913]

[150] Xiang X, Jiang Y, Ni Y, *et al.* Catechol-O-methyltransferase polymorphisms do not play a significant role in pain perception in male Chinese Han population. Physiol Genomics 2012; 44(5): 318-28.
[http://dx.doi.org/10.1152/physiolgenomics.00162.2011] [PMID: 22253202]

[151] Martínez-Jauand M, Sitges C, Rodríguez V, *et al.* Pain sensitivity in fibromyalgia is associated with catechol-O-methyltransferase (COMT) gene. Eur J Pain 2013; 17(1): 16-27.
[http://dx.doi.org/10.1002/j.1532-2149.2012.00153.x] [PMID: 22528689]

[152] Skouen JS, Smith AJ, Warrington NM, *et al.* Genetic variation in the beta-2 adrenergic receptor is associated with chronic musculoskeletal complaints in adolescents. Eur J Pain 2012; 16(9): 1232-42.
[http://dx.doi.org/10.1002/j.1532-2149.2012.00131.x] [PMID: 22416031]

[153] Finan PH, Zautra AJ, Davis MC, Lemery-Chalfant K, Covault J, Tennen H. COMT moderates the relation of daily maladaptive coping and pain in fibromyalgia. Pain 2011; 152(2): 300-7.
[http://dx.doi.org/10.1016/j.pain.2010.10.024] [PMID: 21130573]

[154] Matsuda JB, Barbosa FR, Morel LJ, *et al.* Serotonin receptor (5-HT 2A) and catechol--methyltransferase (COMT) gene polymorphisms: triggers of fibromyalgia? Rev Bras Reumatol 2010; 50(2): 141-9.
[http://dx.doi.org/10.1590/S0482-50042010000200004] [PMID: 21125150]

[155] Barbosa FR, Matsuda JB, Mazucato M, *et al.* Influence of catechol-O-methyltransferase (COMT) gene polymorphisms in pain sensibility of Brazilian fibromialgia patients. Rheumatol Int 2012; 32(2): 427-30.
[http://dx.doi.org/10.1007/s00296-010-1659-z] [PMID: 21120493]

[156] Vossen H, Kenis G, Rutten B, van Os J, Hermens H, Lousberg R. The genetic influence on the cortical processing of experimental pain and the moderating effect of pain status. PLoS One 2010; 5(10): e13641.
[http://dx.doi.org/10.1371/journal.pone.0013641] [PMID: 21049025]

[157] Dai F, Belfer I, Schwartz CE, *et al.* Association of catechol-O-methyltransferase genetic variants with outcome in patients undergoing surgical treatment for lumbar degenerative disc disease. Spine J 2010; 10(11): 949-57.
[http://dx.doi.org/10.1016/j.spinee.2010.07.387] [PMID: 20863768]

[158] Hocking LJ, Smith BH, Jones GT, Reid DM, Strachan DP, Macfarlane GJ. Genetic variation in the beta2-adrenergic receptor but not catecholamine-O-methyltransferase predisposes to chronic pain: results from the 1958 British Birth Cohort Study. Pain 2010; 149(1): 143-51.
[http://dx.doi.org/10.1016/j.pain.2010.01.023] [PMID: 20167428]

[159] Cohen H, Neumann L, Glazer Y, Ebstein RP, Buskila D. The relationship between a common catechol-O-methyltransferase (COMT) polymorphism val(158) met and fibromyalgia. Clin Exp Rheumatol 2009; 27(5) (Suppl. 56): S51-6.
[PMID: 20074440]

[160] McLean SA, Diatchenko L, Lee YM, *et al.* Catechol O-methyltransferase haplotype predicts immediate musculoskeletal neck pain and psychological symptoms after motor vehicle collision. J Pain 2011; 12(1): 101-7.
[http://dx.doi.org/10.1016/j.jpain.2010.05.008] [PMID: 20688576]

[161] Diatchenko L, Slade GD, Nackley AG, *et al.* Genetic basis for individual variations in pain perception and the development of a chronic pain condition. Hum Mol Genet 2005; 14(1): 135-43.
[http://dx.doi.org/10.1093/hmg/ddi013] [PMID: 15537663]

[162] George SZ, Dover GC, Wallace MR, *et al.* Biopsychosocial influence on exercise-induced delayed onset muscle soreness at the shoulder: pain catastrophizing and catechol-o-methyltransferase (COMT) diplotype predict pain ratings. Clin J Pain 2008; 24(9): 793-801.
[http://dx.doi.org/10.1097/AJP.0b013e31817bcb65] [PMID: 18936597]

[163] Vargas-Alarcón G, Fragoso JM, Cruz-Robles D, *et al.* Catechol-O-methyltransferase gene haplotypes in Mexican and Spanish patients with fibromyalgia. Arthritis Res Ther 2007; 9(5): R110.
[http://dx.doi.org/10.1186/ar2316] [PMID: 17961261]

[164] Jensen KB, Lonsdorf TB, Schalling M, Kosek E, Ingvar M. Increased sensitivity to thermal pain following a single opiate dose is influenced by the COMT val(158)met polymorphism. PLoS One 2009; 4(6): e6016.
[http://dx.doi.org/10.1371/journal.pone.0006016] [PMID: 19547755]

[165] Inanir A, Karakus N, Ates O, *et al.* Clinical symptoms in fibromyalgia are associated to catechol-O-methyltransferase (COMT) gene Val158Met polymorphism. Xenobiotica 2014; 44(10): 952-6.
[http://dx.doi.org/10.3109/00498254.2014.913083] [PMID: 24762091]

[166] Dai F, Belfer I, Schwartz CE, *et al.* Association of catechol-O-methyltransferase genetic variants with outcome in patients undergoing surgical treatment for lumbar degenerative disc disease. Spine J 2010; 10(11): 949-57.
[http://dx.doi.org/10.1016/j.spinee.2010.07.387] [PMID: 20863768]

[167] Belfer I, Segall SK, Lariviere WR, *et al.* Pain modality- and sex-specific effects of COMT genetic functional variants. Pain 2013; 154(8): 1368-76.
[http://dx.doi.org/10.1016/j.pain.2013.04.028] [PMID: 23701723]

CHAPTER 5

Non-Pharmacological Treatment Options for Coexisting Chronic Non-Cancer Pain and Substance Use Disorder

Peter Przekop[1,2,*]

[1] *Betty Ford Center, Rancho Mirage, CA 92270, USA*

[2] *Departments of Pediatrics and Psychiatry, Loma Linda University School of Medicine, Loma Linda, CA 92350, USA*

Abstract: Chronic non-cancer pain (CNCP) presents significant challenges to physicians and when combined with co-occurring diseases such as substance use disorder (SUD) the challenge becomes magnified. It is important that the physician realizes that both CNCP and SUD are diseases of the brain, mind, body, and spirit and, therefore, consideration of the whole person and their life experience is essential. In formulating a treatment plan, the physician should remember the cognitive and emotional changes that have occurred as a result of the disease's effect upon the and mind. The proper treatment of the patient should also include treatment of chronic stress and its consequences. The physician should be aware of the alternative modalities such as mind-body, psychosocial, and technology based treatments. Many are available to the patient locally and can also be accessed through the internet. Physicians who treat complex CNCP patients should begin to implement these modalities in a comprehensive treatment plan that restores balance to the patient with CNCP and SUD and allows the patient to become an active participant in their care.

Keywords: Brain, Chronic non-cancer pain, Cognition, Mind-body therapy Nociceptor, Substance use disorder.

* **Coresponding author Peter Przekop:** Betty Ford Center, 39000 Bob Hope Drive, Rancho Mirage, CA 92270, USA; E-mail: pprzekop@llu.edu

Puneetpal Singh (Ed.)

INTRODUCTION

Many physicians are faced with difficult challenges when treating chronic non-cancer pain (CNCP) and the many occurring processes that it is associated with. This situation has become somewhat easier since new research that has occurred over the last two decades has made it clear that CNCP is a fundamentally different disease process when compared to acute pain. Indeed, CNCP is a disease process in which the brain has transformed, reorganized, and has become capable of generating pain spontaneously [1 - 3]. It is now clear that CNCP is very complex which explains why the simplistic Cartesian approach in which a peripheral nociceptive input is treated is ineffective [4 - 6]. Effective treatments must consider the mind, brain, body, and spirit [7]. The current lack of such treatments has left many physicians in a difficult position especially those who treat patients with CNCP and co-occurring substance use disorder (SUD) [8].

This apparent gap in treatment options can be filled by alternative treatment options which range from mind-body therapies, to psychosocial treatments, to technology based therapies, all of which can offer healing to complex CNCP patients. These treatments are effective and popular because they support healing as opposed to chronic disease management, add balance, and well-being, and are devoid of adverse effects [7]. An estimated 62% of Americans take advantage of them [9, 10].

The Scope of the CNCP Problem

CNCP confers considerable suffering to many and is currently at epidemic levels [11]. An estimated half of all patients with SUD also have CNCP [12]. Patients with CNCP and SUD are very difficult to treat with conventional Western medicine, generally pharmacologic methods because they seek help for much more than just physical pain [13, 14]. Most suffer from co-occurring anxiety, symptoms of depression, chronic stress, multiple problems, and the culmination of adversity they have and do suffer from [15]. Most of these patients will be improperly selected for chronic opioid therapy in an attempt to relieve their suffering. However, historically, they have been excluded from opioid clinical trials [16] and thus, there is virtually no evidence to guide opioid-based treatment choices [17]. To complicate matters, it is essential that CNCP is adequately treated in these patients because 60% of them report that pain significantly contributes to the development of SUD [18]. Moreover, effective treatment has been shown to normalize the changes which occur in the brain as a result of CNCP [19].

The Patient with CNCP and SUD

When approaching the patient with CNCP and SUD it is important for the physician to realize that the brain, mind, body, and spirit have been transformed and reorganized. The structural, functional, and connectivity changes of the brain have been extensively reported [20 - 22]. The reorganization of neural networks involved in goal-directed behavior, attention, internal surveillance, emotional regulation, and the ability to enjoy natural rewards have all resulted in significant changes [21] in the patient's ability to think, regulate emotions, regulate behavior, and maintain a positive outlook [23, 24].

Patients with CNCP and SUD have biased acquisition and processing of information that distorts thinking and continues to activate and sustain both disease states. The patient has lost attentional control and attention has been captured by the pain signal which makes it difficult to disengage attention from drug related cues. This results in a bias towards pain-related and drug-related cognitions. In addition, self-referential thought focuses on poor health and poor well-being further contributing to a loss of emotional regulation. Therefore, emotions are negatively valanced and thinking is skewed towards prolonged suffering, poor self-efficacy, pain catastrophizing, and fear of future pain [25].

These factors manifest in the patient as increases in the perception of pain and increases in the areas of the body in which the pain manifests. On days in which the above symptoms are especially severe the patient's perception of physical pain worsens. All is exacerbated by increases in acute and chronic stress.

Patients with both CNCP and SUD report high levels of current suffering and 96% of these patients report a history of unresolved adversity [17, 23, 26]. This results in a dysregulated chronic stress response [27, 28]. Patients display poor coping and report a lack of optimism [25]. In approaching these patients all of these factors should be considered [26, 29, 30].

An Approach to the Patient with CNCP and SUD

History of Present Illness (HPI)

In approaching the patient it is important to consider how the patient has changed as a result of CNCP and SUD. The best approach is to consider the whole person and inquire about all factors that are contributing to the patient's suffering [31, 32]. In addition to a comprehensive HPI, ask the patient about the following:

1. What is the patient's coping style (active *vs*. passive)?
2. Ability to access and process emotions?
3. Hope and motivation for change and healing?
4. Fear of attempting new treatments?
5. Perception about the effectiveness of their current treatment?
6. When was the last time that they felt well?
7. How long they have been under stress?
8. Present level of stress, sleep, exercise, and mindful activities?
9. Barriers to change?
10. The patient's sense of self-worth and self-esteem?
11. What they may be contributing to their suffering?
12. Ability to achieve a quiet mind?

Inquire about when the patient began to:

1. Feel anxious,
2. Experience a lack of well-being,
3. Experience bad feelings inside their body.

It may be useful to use a (0-not at all to 10-extreme) scale to rate these questions.

Other Factors

In addition to a comprehensive HPI, obtain a past medical history, social history, family history, and medication list. In accessing medications consider interactions, adverse effects of medications alongwith dependence and addictive potential.

Physical Exam

A complete physical exam is important with special attention to any asymmetrical findings in bulk, muscle strength, reflexes, and sensations.

Palpate muscle groups for signs of spasms, reduced range of motion, allodynia, and hyperalgesia.

Assess allodynia by having the patient sit in a chair. Use your index and middle fingers to apply gentle pressure bilaterally to the middle of the trapezius muscles. Determine if minimal pressure is perceived as painful.

Potential Treatments

This section will present non-pharmacologic treatments that can easily be accessed by physicians. They will be divided into mind/body, psychosocial, and technology based treatments.

Movement

Movement therapies are available and effective. Amongst the oldest and most extensively studied are qi gong, tai chi, and yoga. All involve movement, breathing, mindfulness, and the ability to move and focus energy to achieve healing. Each has the ability to help the patient with CNCP to regain a sense of self-efficacy, optimism and improve physical as well as psychological strength.

Internal Qi gong is an ancient method of healing that uses qi (life energy), movement, and a meditative state to promote healing. People who practice qi gong are able to increase qi and promote healing by allowing the body, mind, and spirit to use their innate healing mechanisms. Qi gong has been used in a multi-modal program to help patients with CNCP and SUD [33].

Tai chi (Ultimate Supreme) is a form of exercise that promotes health, from both psychological and physiological perspectives. It is another form of healing that uses movement, breathing, and qi energy. It is a form of martial arts that has been used to help patients with chronic pain [34].

Yoga is a series of spiritual and physical beliefs that are used to promote awareness and healing. Yoga utilizes breathing, exercise, and posture to promote health. Numerous studies have shown the benefits of yoga in helping patients with CNCP [35].

Martial Arts is a viable option in treating patients. The practice is intended to promote healing through mindfulness, meditative states, qi energy, and a disciplined lifestyle. Martial arts classes are probably the easiest to access, but physicians should proceed with caution to be certain that the instructors are promoting the art and not the fighting techniques.

Other forms of exercise, movement, and stretching have been explored to help people with CNCP and positive results are reported [36]. It is best to explore the type of movement before it is recommended to the patient.

Energy Therapies

Therapeutic touch/healing touch began with the ancient technique of laying on hands. The goal of this technique is to balance the vital energy fields that exist in the body. The idea is that the practitioner's healing touch can positively influence health. A limited number of studies have shown positive results for CNCP [37].

Reiki is a Japanese term that translates to "universal life energy." Reiki practitioners believe that they channel spiritual energy. Through this process the patients gain spiritual healing. Reiki has been shown to impact pain positively [12].

External qi gong practitioners can move energy and use it to help patients heal. Practitioners are able to channel their energy, the patient's energy, and universal healing energy. Qi activates the natural ability of the mind, body, brain, and spirit to heal. External qi gong has been used to treat patients with CNCP and SUD [31].

Acupuncture and acupressure are techniques that increase the flow of qi in the body. Acupuncture uses needles at specific acupuncture points while acupressure uses pressure applied at specific points. Both have been used extensively to help people with CNCP [38].

Psychosocial Treatments

These treatments are designed to motivate the patient to change while increasing insight about the contribution of cognitions, emotions, and behaviors to illness.

Motivational interviewing is a patient-centered approach that offers encouragement to the patient to undergo change of behaviors through choice and empowerment. The idea is to help the patient to realize that a targeted behavioral change is of benefit and can help eliminate maladaptive thoughts and behaviors that lead to poor choices and reduced self-efficacy [39].

Cognitive restructuring is based on the idea that positive adaptive thoughts lead to increase optimism, mood, adaptive behaviors, and a healthy lifestyle. The treatment involves increasing the patient's awareness of cognitions and how to recognize those cognitions for their positive or negative effects upon behavior and health. The patients are encouraged to replace any maladaptive thoughts with adaptive ones.

Cognitive-behavioral therapy (CBT) is a broad category of different treatment regimens that include cognitive therapy as a primary component. CBT emphasizes changes in behavior. It includes coping skills, relaxation skills, pacing/activity/rest cycling, exercise, and enjoyment [26].

Acceptance-based cognitive therapy (ACT) is a modification of CBT that uses acceptance techniques that emphasize a separation of self from thoughts and feelings in relation to the pain experience. The treatment emphasis is cognitive flexibility and the moment to moment non-judgmental attentiveness to the pain experience. Acceptance based therapies include acceptance and commitment therapy, contextual cognitive behavioral therapy, and mindfulness-based cognitive therapy [16, 38].

Operant training is based on the belief that behaviors are repeated because they are re-enforced. Behaviors that are followed by negative re-enforcers should decrease in frequency. The idea is that if pain persists and becomes chronic there are behavioral re-enforcers that are keeping it present [32].

Hypnosis treatment is a modality that has the patient focus on their attention or on a single sensory experience. Suggestions are then, offered that encourage changes in thoughts, emotions, attention, sensory experience, and behaviors. Finally, a number of post-hypnotic suggestions are offered. Hypnosis can reduce the patient's pain experience [40].

Relaxation training teaches patients how to achieve relaxation. There are a number of techniques such as progressive muscle relaxation, biofeedback, and autogenic training. All of these have been shown to reduce CNCP [2].

Mindfulness/meditation is an essential treatment for CNCP patients. There are a number of meditation and mindfulness techniques that are able to quiet the mind and reduce judgment and suffering.

Other Treatments

Chiropractic treatments use high velocity and low velocity forces to realign structural abnormalities in the body. Chiropractic treatments are comparable to conventional treatments for CNCP [25].

Osteopathic manipulation/cranial sacral therapy are osteopathic techniques that use the body's natural ability to heal while restoring blood flow and structural integrity to the body. Cranial sacral therapy attempts to restore the body's natural rhythm and enhance healing. Both techniques have been used to help patients with CNCP and SUD [33].

Massage therapy involves a trained masseuse using their hands in a therapeutic way to promote healing. There are many different styles of massage that range from very gentle to deep tissue techniques. Massage is generally used as an adjunctive therapy to promote muscle relaxation, stress reduction, and to promote a silent mind. Several studies have shown that massage improves CNCP [41].

Pulsed electromagnetic fields are produced by using generator units. These units stimulate the patient's tissues to promote blood flow and healing. They have been shown to reduce headaches significantly [42].

Cranial electro therapy stimulation involves the steady delivery of low output electrical current to the skin to painful areas. It is hypothesized that the electrical current engages neuro- physiological and neuro-chemical systems to relieve pain. Favorable outcomes have been reported using this technique [43].

Transcutaneous electrical nerve stimulation (TENS) is a self-contained unit that can be applied to the skin. It is thought to work by reducing nociceptive input and by activating central inhibition pain pathways. Multiple studies have shown its effectiveness [44].

Transcranial magnetic stimulation (TMS) uses an electromagnet to generate a magnetic field. The unit is placed over the scalp and can result in small sustained reductions in electrical activity in the area of the brain that is stimulated. It has been used successfully for the treatment of CNCP [45].

Treating the patient using alternative techniques

In considering a treatment plan for the patient the physician has the opportunity to consider the whole person and all of the potential factors that are contributing to the patient's suffering. A treatment plan should include an evaluation of the factors that the patient may be contributing to their continued suffering. This will aid the physician in formulating a plan that considers the whole person and begins to engage the patient as an active participant in their care. Patients with CNCP and SUD are often complex and can present a number of challenges that cannot be addressed by medications only. It is important to remember that the body, mind, brain, and spirit all have the inherent ability to heal. From this perspective, the physician's job is to integrate a full range of treatment options available to aid this patient. The patient's brain, mind, body and spirit are all out of balance and must be brought back into balance.

Pain is a conscious experience that has a dramatic influence upon awareness. Consciousness can be thought of as an ongoing narrative (the story of the world that you perceive) and the autobiographical narrative (story of you in the world). Generally, the patient's narrative becomes significantly altered by CNCP and SUD. It is biased towards a negative outlook, a focus upon negative emotions, a lack of well-being, and poor self-efficacy. The patient is chronically stressed, often has insomnia, maladaptive thinking, emotional dysregulation, and anxiety. The first step in helping the patient is to establish a trusting relationship. The concept of whole-person care and its benefits should be thoroughly explained. The patient should be told that it is important for them to be an active participant in the treatment.

The patient's treatment should include a psychosocial component. It would be best when they could engage in group therapy that has a focus on CNCP. This allows them to express their feelings, change their thinking, and address their adversity in a safe and non-judgmental environment. It will also allow them to relate to the experience of others in the group and give them a sense that they are not alone in their struggle.

A mindfulness component can help patients begin to achieve a quiet mind and allow them to begin to reduce their chronic stress. A movement component could help the patient learn to move in a pain-free way, move energy, and achieve a quiet mind. Patients often benefit from an energy therapy such as acupuncture, external qi gong or reiki. As patients learn these treatments they can begin to practice them at home. This leads to increased self-confidence, optimism, and self-efficacy. Patients should always have their medications carefully reviewed to determine if they are contributing to increased pain, anxiety or symptoms of depression.

When approaching the patient, it is important for the physician to begin to gain a sense of how much willingness they have to change and to become an active participant in their recovery. Initially, patients may be highly resistant to change and for active participation. The physician can help them gain important insight by pointing out the reasons why their current plan is ineffective. It may be helpful to give patients examples of others who have become actively involved in their treatment and have changed their lives and reduced suffering. It will be important that patients understand that there is a way to reduce their suffering and allow them to gain balance and a quiet mind.

The patients should be asked if they have previously engaged in alternative treatments. It might be easiest to encourage them to try an energy technique such as reiki or external qi gong. They should be encouraged to consider a qi gong or a yoga class as a form of movement. These movement techniques are also available through the Internet at no cost, so if payment is an issue this may be an option. The goal of treatment is to teach the patient techniques to reduce stress, change their thinking, and begin to understand what they must change to their suffering. They should be encouraged to begin a daily routine of practicing the treatment techniques they have learned. This will allow them to begin self-directed healing. When the patient begins to experience positive results it will serve as motivation. This will also help them to engage in treatment for SUD such as twelve-step recovery.

The physician should become aware of the services that are available to patients in their area. The physician should consider studying and becoming proficient in some of the recommended therapies. This can add to the patient's personal program of self-care while allowing the physician to lend first hand expertise to the patient. Once the physician becomes knowledgeable about alternative options and realizes their value, it will allow him to begin to integrate a full range of therapies into their patient's treatment plan. This will lead to improved care and more options that will help difficult patients to reduce suffering and improve their lives.

Final Considerations

Patients who are dependent upon medications or substances will derive sub-optimal benefit from non-pharmacologic treatments. In order to balance and enhance the brain, mind, body, and spirit it is necessary to be drug free. No patient is too old or too ill to engage in any of these treatment modalities. It is necessary to inform the patient that they should enter at a level in which they feel comfortable. Many modalities can begin from a chair or even bed. Many non-pharmacologic treatments can be obtained on the internet, at a bookstore, or by mail order. Mindfulness, movement therapy, pain blogs or internet groups are all available online.

CONFLICT OF INTEREST

The authors confirm that they have no conflict of interest to declare for this publication.

ACKNOWLEDGEMENTS

Declared none.

REFERENCES

[1] Vowles KE, Witkiewitz K, Sowden G, Ashworth J. Acceptance and commitment therapy for chronic pain: evidence of mediation and clinically significant change following an abbreviated interdisciplinary program of rehabilitation. J Pain 2014; 15(1): 101-13. [http://dx.doi.org/10.1016/j.jpain.2013.10.002] [PMID: 24373572]

[2] Williams DA. Psychological and behavioural therapies in fibromyalgia and related syndromes. Best Pract Res Clin Rheumatol 2003; 17(4): 649-65. [http://dx.doi.org/10.1016/S1521-6942(03)00034-2] [PMID: 12849717]

[3] Brevik H. World Health Organization supports global effort to relieve chronic pain 2015. Retrieved from: http//www.who,int/mediacentre/news/releases/2004/pr70/en/print.html

[4] Barry DT, Pilver C, Potenza MN, Desai RA. Prevalence and psychiatric correlates of pain interference among men and women in the general population. J Psychiatr Res 2012; 46(1): 118-27. [http://dx.doi.org/10.1016/j.jpsychires.2011.09.004] [PMID: 21944430]

[5] Odding E, Valkenburg HA, Algra D, Vandenouweland FA, Grobbee DE, Hofman A. Associations of radiological osteoarthritis of the hip and knee with locomotor disability in the Rotterdam Study. Ann Rheum Dis 1998; 57(4): 203-8. [http://dx.doi.org/10.1136/ard.57.4.203] [PMID: 9709175]

[6] Gaukroger S. Descartes: An Intellectual Biography. Oxford: Clarendon Press 1995.

[7] Przekop P, Haviland MG, Przekop A. Characteristics of Patients Admitted to an Inpatient Program for Chronic Pain and Substance Use Disorder. meeting of the American Academy of Pain Management. Phoenix Arizona. 2014.

[8] Pohl M, Smith L. Chronic pain and addiction: challenging co-occurring disorders. J Psychoactive Drugs 2012; 44(2): 119-24. [http://dx.doi.org/10.1080/02791072.2012.684621] [PMID: 22880539]

[9] Nahin RL, Barnes PM, Stussman BJ, Bloom B. Costs of complementary and alternative medicine (CAM) and frequency of visits to CAM practitioners: United States, 2007. Hyattsville MD National Center for Health Statistics 2009; 8: 1-15.

[10] Barnes PM, Powell-Griner E, McFann K, Nahin RL. Complementary and alternative medicine use among adults: United States, 2002. Adv Data 2004; (343): 1-19. [PMID: 15188733]

[11] Dominick CH, Blyth FM, Nicholas MK. Unpacking the burden: understanding the relationships between chronic pain and comorbidity in the general population. Pain 2012; 153(2): 293-304. [http://dx.doi.org/10.1016/j.pain.2011.09.018] [PMID: 22071318]

[12] Miles P. Preliminary report on the use of Reiki HIV-related pain and anxiety. Altern Ther Health Med 2003; 9(2): 36. [PMID: 12652881]

[13] Pade PA, Cardon KE, Hoffman RM, Geppert CM. Prescription opioid abuse, chronic pain, and primary care: a Co-occurring Disorders Clinic in the chronic disease model. J Subst Abuse Treat 2012; 43(4): 446-50.
[http://dx.doi.org/10.1016/j.jsat.2012.08.010] [PMID: 22980449]

[14] Melzack R. From the gate to the neuromatrix. Pain 1999; 82 (Suppl. 6): S121-6.
[http://dx.doi.org/10.1016/S0304-3959(99)00145-1] [PMID: 10491980]

[15] Kroenke K, Outcalt S, Krebs E, *et al.* Association between anxiety, health-related quality of life and functional impairment in primary care chronic pain patients. Gen Hosp Psychiatry 2013; 359-65.
[http://dx.doi.org/10.1016/j.genhosppsych.2013.03.020] [PMID: 23639186]

[16] Howe CQ, Sullivan MD. The missing 'P' in pain management: how the current opioid epidemic highlights the need for psychiatric services in chronic pain care. Gen Hosp Psychiatry 2014; 36(1): 99-104.
[http://dx.doi.org/10.1016/j.genhosppsych.2013.10.003] [PMID: 24211157]

[17] Reuben DB, Alvanzo AA, Ashikaga T, *et al.* National Institutes of Health Pathways to Prevention Workshop: the role of opioids in the treatment of chronic pain. Ann Intern Med 2015; 162(4): 295-300.
[http://dx.doi.org/10.7326/M14-2775] [PMID: 25581341]

[18] Cicero TJ, Lynskey M, Todorov A, Inciardi JA, Surratt HL. Co-morbid pain and psychopathology in males and females admitted to treatment for opioid analgesic abuse. Pain 2008; 139(1): 127-35.
[http://dx.doi.org/10.1016/j.pain.2008.03.021] [PMID: 18455314]

[19] Seminowicz DA, Wideman TH, Naso L, *et al.* Effective treatment of chronic low back pain in humans reverses abnormal brain anatomy and function. J Neurosci 2011; 31(20): 7540-50.
[http://dx.doi.org/10.1523/JNEUROSCI.5280-10.2011] [PMID: 21593339]

[20] Becker S, Gandhi W, Schweinhardt P. Cerebral interactions of pain and reward and their relevance for chronic pain. Neurosci Lett 2012; 520(2): 182-7.
[http://dx.doi.org/10.1016/j.neulet.2012.03.013] [PMID: 22440855]

[21] Apkarian AV, Baliki MN, Geha PY. Towards a theory of chronic pain. Prog Neurobiol 2009; 87(2): 81-97.
[http://dx.doi.org/10.1016/j.pneurobio.2008.09.018] [PMID: 18952143]

[22] Turner JA, Chapman CR. Psychological interventions for chronic pain: a critical review. I. Relaxation training and biofeedback. Pain 1982; 12(1): 1-21.
[http://dx.doi.org/10.1016/0304-3959(82)90167-1] [PMID: 7036049]

[23] Meulders A, Vansteenwegen D, Vlaeyen JW. Women, but not men, report increasingly more pain during repeated (un)predictable painful electrocutaneous stimulation: Evidence for mediation by fear of pain. Pain 2012; 153(5): 1030-41.
[http://dx.doi.org/10.1016/j.pain.2012.02.005] [PMID: 22401700]

[24] Tracey I. Imaging pain. Br J Anaesth 2008; 101(1): 32-9.
[http://dx.doi.org/10.1093/bja/aen102] [PMID: 18556697]

[25] Cherkin DC, Eisenberg D, Sherman KJ, *et al.* Randomized trial comparing traditional Chinese medical acupuncture, therapeutic massage, and self-care education for chronic low back pain. Arch Intern Med

2001; 161(8): 1081-8.
[http://dx.doi.org/10.1001/archinte.161.8.1081] [PMID: 11322842]

[26] Young Casey C, Greenberg MA, Nicassio PM, Harpin RE, Hubbard D. Transition from acute to chronic pain and disability: a model including cognitive, affective, and trauma factors. Pain 2008; 134(1-2): 69-79.
[http://dx.doi.org/10.1016/j.pain.2007.03.032] [PMID: 17504729]

[27] Gold PW. The organization of the stress system and its dysregulation in depressive illness. Mol Psychiatry 2015; 20(1): 32-47.
[http://dx.doi.org/10.1038/mp.2014.163] [PMID: 25486982]

[28] Koob GF. Addiction as a reward deficit and stress surfeit disorder. Front Psychiatry 2013; 4: 72.
[http://dx.doi.org/10.3389/fpsyt.2013.00072] [PMID: 23914176]

[29] Przekop P, Przekop A, Haviland MG. Perception of chronic non cancer pain patients prescribed and not prescribed opioids. Poster Presentation American Academy of Neurology Annual Meeting Washington, DC. 2015.

[30] Gatchel RJ, Peng YB, Peters ML, Fuchs PN, Turk DC. The biopsychosocial approach to chronic pain: scientific advances and future directions. Psychol Bull 2007; 133(4): 581-624.
[http://dx.doi.org/10.1037/0033-2909.133.4.581] [PMID: 17592957]

[31] Przekop P, Przekop A, Haviland MG, Riggs M. Neuro-cognitive-enhancement for the treatment of chronic pain. J Bodyw Mov Ther 2010; 14: e334-5.
[http://dx.doi.org/10.1016/j.jbmt.2009.10.003]

[32] Elman I, Borsook D, Volkow ND. Pain and suicidality: insights from reward and addiction neuroscience. Prog Neurobiol 2013; 109: 1-27.
[http://dx.doi.org/10.1016/j.pneurobio.2013.06.003] [PMID: 23827972]

[33] Przekop PR, Tulgan H, Przekop A, DeMarco WJ, Campbell N, Kisiel S. The implementation of an osteopathic clinic at an allopathic teaching hospital: a research based experience. J Am Osteopath Assoc 2003; 103: 343-550.
[PMID: 14686624]

[34] Peng PW. Tai chi and chronic pain. Reg Anesth Pain Med 2012; 37(4): 372-82.
[http://dx.doi.org/10.1097/AAP.0b013e31824f6629] [PMID: 22609642]

[35] Cramer H, Lauche R, Hohmann C, *et al.* Randomized-controlled trial comparing yoga and home-based exercise for chronic neck pain. Clin J Pain 2013; 29(3): 216-23.
[http://dx.doi.org/10.1097/AJP.0b013e318251026c] [PMID: 23249655]

[36] Nijs J, Lluch Girbés E, Lundberg M, Malfliet A, Sterling M. Exercise therapy for chronic musculoskeletal pain: Innovation by altering pain memories. Man Ther 2015; 20(1): 216-20.
[http://dx.doi.org/10.1016/j.math.2014.07.004] [PMID: 25090974]

[37] Keller E, Bzdek VM. Effects of therapeutic touch on tension headache pain. Nurs Res 1986; 35(2): 101-6.
[PMID: 3633503]

[38] Witt CM, Jena S, Brinkhaus B, Liecker B, Wegscheider K, Willich SN. Acupuncture for patients with chronic neck pain. Pain 2006; 125(1-2): 98-106.

[http://dx.doi.org/10.1016/j.pain.2006.05.013] [PMID: 16781068]

[39] Miller WR, Rollnick S. Motivational interviewing: preparing people for change. New York: Guilford Press 2002.

[40] Jensen M, Pattersen DR. Hypnosis in therelief of pain and pain disorders. In: Nash MR, Barnier A, Eds. Contemporary hypnosis research. Oxford University Press 2008; pp. 508-33.

[41] Hernandez-Reif M, Field T, Krasnegor J, Theakston H. Lower back pain is reduced and range of motion increased after massage therapy. Int J Neurosci 2001; 106(3-4): 131-45. [http://dx.doi.org/10.3109/00207450109149744] [PMID: 11264915]

[42] Sherman RA, Acosta NM, Robson L. Treatment of migraine with pulsing electromagnetic fields: a double-blind, placebo-controlled study. Headache 1999; 39(8): 567-75. [http://dx.doi.org/10.1046/j.1526-4610.1999.3908567.x] [PMID: 11279973]

[43] Hefferman M. The effect of variable microcurrents on EEG spectrum and pain control. Canadian J of Cl Med 1997; 4: 4-11.

[44] Dailey DL, Rakel BA, Vance CG, *et al.* Transcutaneous electrical nerve stimulation reduces pain, fatigue and hyperalgesia while restoring central inhibition in primary fibromyalgia. Pain 2013; 154(11): 2554-62.
[http://dx.doi.org/10.1016/j.pain.2013.07.043] [PMID: 23900134]

[45] Dall'Agnol L, Medeiros LF, Torres IL, *et al.* Repetitive transcranial magnetic stimulation increases the corticospinal inhibition and the brain-derived neurotrophic factor in chronic myofascial pain syndrome: an explanatory double-blinded, randomized, sham-controlled trial. J Pain 2014; 15(8): 845-55.
[http://dx.doi.org/10.1016/j.jpain.2014.05.001] [PMID: 24865417]

CHAPTER 6

MicroRNAs: The Tiny Robust Players Unraveling the Multifaceted Channels of Pain

Yogita K. Adlakha*

Cellular and Molecular Neuroscience, National Brain Research Centre, Manesar-122051, India

Abstract: Pain is a debilitating condition which is the leading cause of cognitive, mood and anxiety disorders. It is one of the major medical burdens on human health which obstructs the quality life of a person as the appropriate therapeutic solution is not available. Due to advancement of new genomic technologies, it is now possible to view genome wide changes during chronic pain in different cell types from the somato-sensory system to the neurons in central nervous system. Tremendous research over recent years has enlightened the magical potential of small non-coding RNAs, mainly microRNAs in modulating numerous pathophysiological processes including proliferation, apoptosis and oncogenesis. They target a wide range of molecules and refine their protein output and thus, fine tune distinct cellular processes including pain signaling. Recently, animal models depicting inflammatory and neuropathic pain and patient subjects complaining distress due to pain have shown deregulations of miRNAs in affected tissues and systemic circulation. Although various painful conditions *viz.* spinal cord injury, peripheral nerve injury, cancer and inflammatory diseases have been recognized with genome-wide changes in microRNA signatures, yet the gene regulatory networks underlying pathological significance of individual microRNAs are sparsely studied. Hence, this chapter summarizes the latest findings addressing the role of microRNAs in various inflammatory or neuropathic pain conditions. How can miRNA research be expedited in revealing new aspects of pain pathophysiology is also addressed. The chapter also uncovers the novel potentials of miRNAs as well as roadblocks in the path of miRNA based anti-nociceptive therapies.

Keywords: DRG, miRNA, Nociceptive pathway, Pain, Spinal cord, TG.

* **Coresponding author Yogita K. Adlakha:** Cellular and Molecular Neuroscience, National Brain Research Centre, Manesar-122051, India; E-mail: yogita@nbrc.ac.in

INTRODUCTION

Although pain is one of the fundamental alarming systems of the body yet chronic pain may devastate the quality of one's life, leading to disturbances in the cognitive and emotional functions. Thus, human disorders associated with the chronic pain including osteoarthritis (OA), post-herpetic neuralgia, diabetic polyneuropathy and migraine represent a large socioeconomic burden. Although recent research has provided fundamental insights into pathological pain, yet effective therapeutic treatments are least available till date. In recent years, accumulating reports have introduced a novel entity in pain that is known as microRNAs (miRNAs) for being small, functional non-coding RNAs in nature that have been playing an instrumental role in regulating pain-processing in various pain settings ranging from experimental models to clinical pain disorders [1 - 4]. These studies have provided the basic understanding for the development of microRNA therapeutics for the treatment of pathological chronic pain in future. The main objective of this chapter is to discuss various implications of miRNAs in pain and to explore ways to expedite the miRNA research in pain pathophysiology. Attention has also been paid to exploring opportunities for the development of miRNAs as a therapy for chronic pain.

Pain

Pain is such an unpleasant feeling which cannot be described in words. It is an obnoxious sensation that is not only associated with sensory experience due to actual or potential tissue damage but also with the elements which alter cognitive and emotional circuitry [5]. Pain can be categorized into two types depending upon the length of stimulus: acute and chronic. Acute pain lasts till the applied stimulus and resolves promptly, thus functions as a central alarming system for the body and protects from damage [6]. However, chronic pain is devastating and outlasts the period of initial injury and thus reduces patient's quality of life. Therefore, there is an urgent call for effective clinical intervention for such unfortunate pain. However, till date, therapeutic solutions are distant from sight due to the hindrance by large numbers of mediators and signaling pathways in the etiology of pain and presence of functional redundancy between them [6]. Further, pain can be divided into two groups depending upon the type of stimuli:

Nociceptive and Neuropathic pain. Nociceptive pain is initiated by signals from damaged tissues or injury which get transferred through peripheral nerves to the brain *via* the spinal cord. This type of pain works as an alerting system for the organism and prepares organism against potential damage. Mostly back, leg and arm pains are nociceptive pains. However, aberrations in somatosensory system can cause damage or disease in the nervous system which is the root cause of neuropathic pain [7]. Chronic neuropathic pain is completely pathological and does not have beneficial aspect. This pain occurs after a stroke or after cutting of nerves and include shingles and diabetic peripheral neuropathy.

The nociceptive pain signaling initiates upon the detection of a nociceptive stimulus by nociceptors. These nociceptors are the primary neurons that have their cell bodies in dorsal root ganglion (DRG) or trigeminal ganglion (TG). However, their peripheral axons sense this stimulus and send this information to DRG or TG *via* their cell bodies. The information is relayed from DRG or TG to the spinal or medullary dorsal horn *via* primary sensory neurons to secondary neurons [5]. Interaction between excitatory and inhibitory inter neurons, glial cells and descending axons from the brainstem form the complex circuits in the dorsal horn, and then process this information and relay the processed information to the higher brain areas which are mainly involved in pain sensation and associated emotions [8, 9]. Somatosensory cortices, prefrontal cortex, amygdala, insular cortex and anterior cingulate cortex form higher brain areas where pain is perceived and sensory and emotional processing of pain occurs [10]. Thus, chronic pain can negatively affect important brain functions including cognition and mood and hence, it is also associated with mood, comorbid cognitive and anxiety disorders [11].

MicroRNA

MicroRNAs (miRNAs) are the small, non-coding pieces of RNA, which were once misunderstood as cellular detritus, have now popped up as master players in the regulation of gene expression in the past decade. MiRNAs comprise a novel class of endogenous, evolutionarily conserved, non-coding single-stranded RNAs of ~19-25 nucleotides in length which mainly operate at post-transcriptional level. They were first discovered in *Caenorhabditis elegans* and since then they have made their presence in both plants and animals [12, 13]. The first pioneer miRNA named lin-4 was identified in 1993 by two independent research groups in *Caenorhabditis elegans* and was reported to control developmental timings [14, 15]. It was only after seven years that another miRNA named let-7 (lethal-7) was discovered as a regulator of the temporal fate specification during development in *C. elegans* [16]. Thanks to the high throughput sequencing technology that thousands of miRNAs have been exposed these days. Recent research has illuminated their role in plethora of cellular and pathophysiological processes including embryonic development, apoptosis, proliferation, differentiation, metabolism, stress responses and inflammation [17 - 23]. Their fundamental influence on several physiological processes renders them master small molecules playing around inside the cells and any disruption in their biogenesis or functional pathways cause severe diseases including cardiovascular diseases [24], cancer [25, 26], neurodegenerative diseases [27], diabetes [28], AIDS [29], chronic hepatitis [30] and CNS injuries [31].

MiRNAs preferentially bind to the 3′ untranslated regions (3′ UTRs) [32, 33] or, occasionally, the 5′UTRs [34, 35] or coding regions [36 - 38] of their target mRNAs and disrupt the expression and function of their target. The fate of target mRNA depends upon the degree of complementation between seed sequence of miRNA and 3′UTR of its target gene. Degradation of target mRNA is generally favored by complete complementation whereas inhibition of translation is seen during partial complementation in mammals [32, 39, 40]. Further, reports suggest that single miRNA can fine tune the gene regulatory networks by targeting several genes simultaneously while several miRNAs can also target a single mRNA in a concerted manner. The latter capacity points towards a method adopted by miRNAs to modulate several biological processes during homeostasis and diseased conditions [41]. The regulation of various biological processes by miRNAs seems to be conserved across different evolutionary classes due to the conserved sequence of miRNAs and their target sites in 3'UTR of mRNAs [42].

Biogenesis of MiRNA and their Mechanism of Action

The location of miRNAs in genome is sculptured very well and can vary from intragenic to intergenic; from introns of long non-coding RNAs to introns or exons of protein-coding genes [43, 44]. For their biogenesis, they can either use host gene's transcriptional machinery or possess their independent transcriptional set up [45]. The transcription of miRNA starts in nucleus just like other protein coding genes by RNA polymerase II/III. Thus, genomic DNA is transcribed into long, primary transcripts known as pri-miRNAs with a 5′ CAP and a 3′ poly (A) tail (Fig. **1**). These primary transcripts vary in length and reach up to a size of few kilobases. A microprocessor complex then chops the pri-miRNAs into smaller transcripts named as precursor miRNAs (pre-miRNA) which are about 70-100 nucleotides long (Fig. **1**). This microprocessor complex is formed by ribonuclease III called Drosha, a RNA binding protein named DGCR8/Pasha and different cofactors which are likely to increase the activity and/or specificity of Drosha [45 - 48]. In case of mammals, Drosha action takes place along with transcription before splicing of host gene's RNA (canonical pathway). However, miRtrons, which represents a class of intronic miRNAs can escape Drosha processing and rather produced by splicing and debranching [49, 50]. For final maturation, these pre-miRNAs are exported out of nucleus by Exportin-5 in a Ran-GTP dependent manner into the cytoplasm [51].

Then, in cytoplasm, two different mechanisms operate to further process these pre-miRNAs into mature form. Either RNase III enzyme Dicer or Ago2 (an Argonaute protein) act to produce the mature, smaller double-stranded RNA (~22 nt) in the form of a duplex from pre-miRNAs [52, 53]. There is remarkable difference in the functioning of Dicer and Ago2. After Dicer chopping, 5′ phosphate groups and two-nucleotide overhangs are added at the 3′ ends of the mature miRNA transcripts. Presence of short stem and miRNA sequence in the stem loop of pre-miRNA defines the criteria for the action of Ago2 which binds and cleaves after the 30th nucleotide. This mature miRNA duplex forms miRISC (miRNA-induced silencing complex) with Argonaute proteins where one strand of mature miRNA duplex designated as "guide strand", usually binds to the 3'UTR of the target gene however, the second strand referred to as the "passenger strand" is released from the miRISC and degraded [54]. The formation and functioning of miRISC also requires several cofactors just like above mentioned two ribonucleases, Drosha and Dicer [55].

These include Argonaute (AGO) proteins and glycine-tryptophan protein of 182 kDa (GW182). The former directly interact with mature strands of miRNAs while the latter act as downstream effectors during repression. This miRISC is then guided by mature miRNA strand to find the potential target sites in the 3′UTR of their target genes (Fig. **1**).

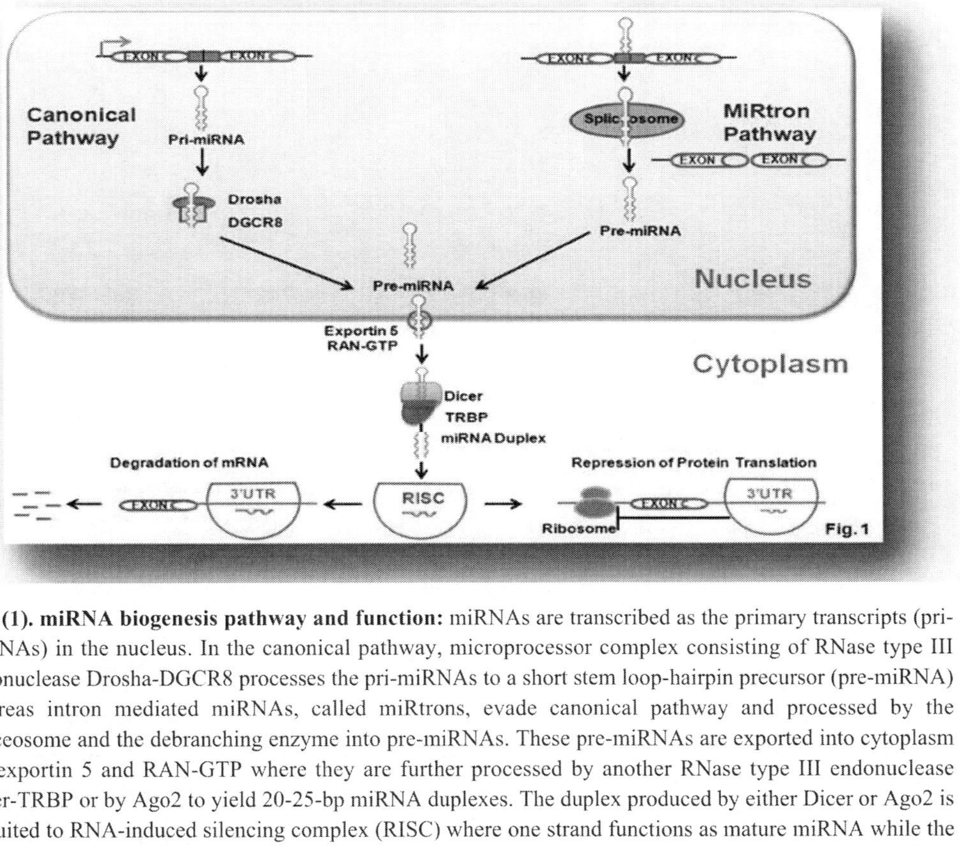

Fig. (1). miRNA biogenesis pathway and function: miRNAs are transcribed as the primary transcripts (pri-miRNAs) in the nucleus. In the canonical pathway, microprocessor complex consisting of RNase type III endonuclease Drosha-DGCR8 processes the pri-miRNAs to a short stem loop-hairpin precursor (pre-miRNA) whereas intron mediated miRNAs, called miRtrons, evade canonical pathway and processed by the spliceosome and the debranching enzyme into pre-miRNAs. These pre-miRNAs are exported into cytoplasm *via* exportin 5 and RAN-GTP where they are further processed by another RNase type III endonuclease Dicer-TRBP or by Ago2 to yield 20-25-bp miRNA duplexes. The duplex produced by either Dicer or Ago2 is recruited to RNA-induced silencing complex (RISC) where one strand functions as mature miRNA while the partner miRNA* strand is preferentially degraded. The mature miRNA produced by these two mechanisms regulates the output of protein-coding genes through diverse mechanisms. The degree of interaction between miRNAs and the 3′ untranslated region (3′ UTR) of protein-coding genes then determines the protein yield. Perfect sequence complementarity between the seed region of miRNA to the target mRNA results in mRNA degradation. Imperfect miRNA seed-mRNA 3’UTR pairing, leads to translational repression.

MiRNA and Target Interaction

The functional relevance of a miRNA can be determined by the function of targeted genes and the effect of miRNA on regulating the translation of a target mRNA. The major factor which contributes to the decision of translational repression of target mRNA or mRNA degradation is the extent of complementary binding between seed region (5′ 2–9 nucleotides 3′) of mature miRNA and 3′UTR of their target mRNA. This binding between miRNA and its target is considered to be Watson-Crick base-pairing [56]. However, the influence of other sequences in UTR besides target site in regulating the miRNA-mRNA interaction has also been observed. Reporter assays have demonstrated that presence of a mere identical site in different UTRs does not guarantee the repression as it has been shown to repress some UTRs but not the others [57]. Thus, it supports the idea that there may be some other UTR features which regulate miRNA-mRNA interactions and also determine the specificity of targeting. One of them could be the enrichment of AU rich nucleotide composition near the binding site which can give way to stronger binding of miRNA to mRNA because of the weaker secondary structure in the vicinity of binding site. Further binding besides the seed region of miRNA defined as other 3′- supplementary and 3′- compensatory binding sites also change the outcome of interaction between miRNA and its target [32]. Further, genome wide analysis indicates that miRNA binding sites are selectively maintained near the ends rather than in the centre of the 3'UTR, especially for longer 3'UTRs [58]. Besides, 3'UTR, miRNAs have also been reported to interact with 5'UTR, intron-exon junctions and CDS (Coding DNA sequence) of their target [34, 36].

Several mechanisms have been suggested underlying the miRNA mediated repression of protein synthesis which include suppression of initiation phase of translation, repression of translation, deadenylation of target followed by degradation of target and long term storage and sequestration of mRNA from ribosomes into P bodies [40, 59]. However, research is still going on to illuminate the detailed mechanisms underlying miRNA mediated repression of their target protein. Further, mRNA decay is supposed to be the most favored mechanism underlying regulation of gene expression by miRNA than translational repression in majority of cases [60]. Besides complementary binding, conventional DNA modifications including epigenetic modifications and cell regulators including transcription factors also modulate the function of miRNAs to a reasonable extent.

Further, some reports also support that pseudogenes also regulate miRNA function by sequestering miRNAs or acting as decoys [61, 62].

Expression Profile of MiRNAs in Different Animal Models of Pain

Unique miRNA expression signatures are not only restricted to specific types of cells, but also indicative of particular disease state. Thus, miRNAs may not only used as diagnostic and prognostic tools, but may also illuminate transcriptional and translational machinery of different chronic pain states [6]. It is well known that several molecules are induced in chronic pain states to orchestrate a particular pain pathway; hence it is assumed that, miRNAs could also articulate the main pathological pathways leading to chronic pain. To find the depth, researchers have performed genome-wide screenings using microarray profiling or deep sequencing to gain insights in to miRNA expression changes in several painful settings, ranging from inflammatory disease to peripheral nerve injury and from spinal cord injury to cancer [5] and illuminated tissue specific deregulated expression of miRNAs in DRG and spinal cord (Fig. **2**). Throughout the pain signaling pathway, modulations in miRNA expression have been determined, in high processing centers such as the emotional circuits to the basal sensory neurons. These studies suggest that dynamic changes occur in miRNA expression which is specific to a particular pain state. Also, temporal alterations in miRNA expression have been observed in DRG and spinal cord after the start of initial events of pain which suggest that the chronic pain is regulated by two distinct phenomena during initiation and maintenance [63, 64]. As changes in miRNA expressions have been shown in the brain areas involved in emotional, cognitive and affective perception of pain which include somatosensory system, prefrontal cortex (PFC) of brain and the limbic system, it is worth to say that during chronic pain, miRNAs may also have crucial roles in other brain deteriorations (Fig. **2**) [5].

Independent studies have shown decrease in the expression of miR-16 and miR-143 in DRG during inflammatory pain but not in case of neuropathic pain and nerve damage respectively (Table **1**) [65, 66]. Further, increase in levels of miR-21 and decrease in levels of miR-7a were observed during late phase of neuropathic pain, however their levels were not changed during inflammatory pain [67, 68]. Additionally, adenovirus associated introduction of miR-7a in sensory neurons of injured DRG in rats, reduced the maintenance of neuropathic pain [68]. Further, up regulation of miR-1a-3p was observed in capsaicin injection, axotomy and bone cancer whereas downregulation was observed upon partial sciatic nerve ligation and CFA injection (Table **1**) [65, 69]. Another study revealed that deletion of miRNA maturing enzyme Dicer in mouse post mitotic damage-sensing neurons in DRG attenuated inflammatory pain and not neuropathic pain [70].

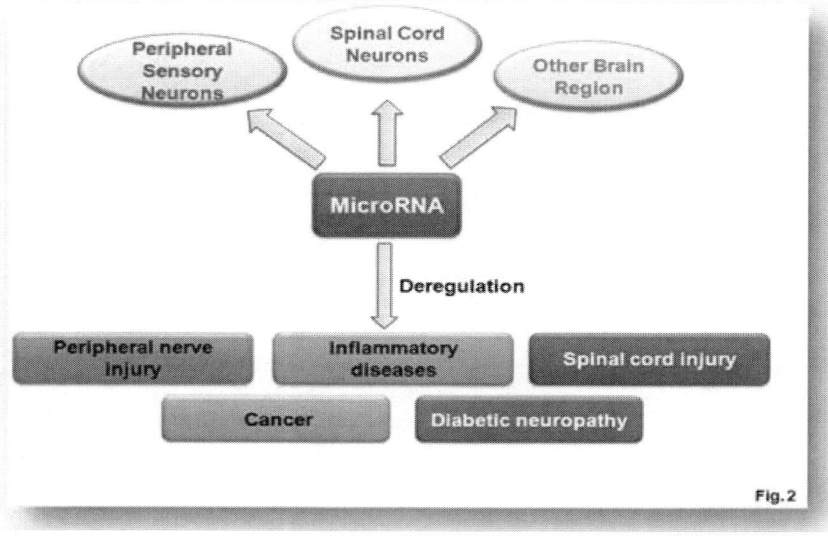

Fig. (2). miRNAs can regulate different components of pain: miRNAs can regulate different components of somatosensory system along the nociceptive pathway starting from primary peripheral neurons to higher central nervous system regions. Deregulation of miRNAs in any of these components can lead to various nociceptive disorders and chronic pain.

Several reports demonstrate the potential of circulating miRNAs to become biomarkers for various diseases. Circulating miRNAs from serum were detected and compared before and after spinal nerve ligation (SNL) surgery in rats. The authors observed down regulation of five miRNAs (hsa-miR-221, hsa-miR-34c, hsa-miR-21, hsa-miR-30a-5p and hsa-miR-206) whereas upregulation of four miRNAs (hsa-miR-31-5p, hsa-miR-133b, hsa-miR-22 and hsa-miRPlus-A1087) after SNL surgery in the serum, further support that during regulation of neuropathic pain, alterations in miRNA levels may play defined roles [71]. Further, miR-30d-5p, miR-125b-5p and miR-379-5p were observed to be differentially regulated in rat DRGs after nerve injury.

Table 1. Table depicts differential expression of number of miRNAs in different regions of somatosensory system during chronic pain.

miRNA	Expression	Pain model	Reference
miRNA-183 cluster (comprising miR-183, miR-182, and miR-96)	Decreased	SNL in mice	[79]
miRNA-183	Decreased	SNL in rat	[124]
miRNA-21	Increased	SNT in rat	[74]
miR-7a	Decreased	SNL in rat	[68]
miR-96	Decreased	CCI in rat	[125]
miR-143	Decreased	SNT in mice	[66]
miR-1, miR-16, miR-206	Increased	SNA in mice	[65]
miR-125b-5p, miR-30d-5p, miR-379-5p	Differentially regulated	SNL in rats genetically segregated to sense high or low neuropathic pain	[72]
miR-183, miR-124a	Decreased	CFA-induced inflammatory muscle pain model in rat	[81]
miR-134	Decreased from 1 to 7 days and increased at 14 days	CFA-induced inflammatory pain model in rat	[126]
miR-183 cluster, miR-146a	Decreased	Knee-joint osteoarthritis (OA) model in rat	[80, 126]
miR-143	Decreased	CFA model in mice	[66]
miR-1, miR-16, miR-206	Decreased	CFA model in mice	[65]
miR-1a-3p, miR-544-3p, miR-34c-5p, and 23 other miRNAs	Increased	Bone metastasis model in mouse	[69]
miR-370-3p, miR-483-3p, miR-291b-5p, and 28 other miRNAs	Decreased	Bone metastasis model in mouse	[69]
miR-1a-3p	Increased	Bone cancer	[69]
miR-137, miR-181a, miR-219-2-3p, and 247 other miRNAs	Differential regulation	Traumatic SCI in rat	[127]
miRNA-203	Decreased	Bilateral CCI in rat	[87]
miR-103	Decreased	SNL in rat	[91]

(Table 1) contd.....

miRNA	Expression	Pain model	Reference
miR-1	Decreased	SNA in mice	[65]
miR-1, miR-124, miR-129-1, miR-129-2	Decreased	SCI in rat	[74]
miR-223	Increased from 6 hours to day 3	SCI in mice	[88]
miR-124a	Decreased from day 1 to 7	SCI in mice	[88]
miR-21	Increased at day 35	SCI in mice	[128]
miR-146a	Decreased	OA in rat	[89]
miR-124a	Decreased from 1 to 24 h, basal levels at 48 h	Intraplantar application of formalin or interleukin-1b (IL-1b) (an inflammatory mediator) in mice	[2] [90],
miR-1, miR-16, miR-206	Increased	CFA in mice	[65]
miR-23b	Decreased	SCI	[129]
miR-195	Increased	SNL	[130]
miR-155, miR-223	Increased	Model of facial inflammatory pain in mouse	[97]
miR-200b, miR-429	Decreased	PNL model of neuropathic pain in mice	[95]
miR-146a, miR-34c, miR-125--5p, miR-1, and others	Decreased	CCI in rat	[93]
let-7 family members, miR-103, and others	Increased	CCI in rat	[93]
miR-let-7a,c,g	Increased	Opioid tolerance	[98]

The authors profiled DRG for miRNA expression from two rat lines which were genetically related but differ in pain response and produce high pain and low pain following spinal nerve injury. Three pro-nociceptive molecules were traced to be the target genes of these miRNAs which include TNF, BDNF and STAT3 and play major roles in pain signaling and pathophysiology [72]. Recently, Gong *et al.* investigated microRNAs profile in the diabetic neuropathic pain (DNP) mice model induced by streptozotocin (STZ) and compared them with vehicle controls. Twenty one miRNAs were found to be significantly up-regulated while other twenty one were down-regulated out of forty two differentially expressed miRNAs. Further, only two differentially expressed miRNAs namely, miR-18--5p and miR-190a-5p displayed similar alterations in DNP tissue both by qRT-

PCR and by microarray analysis. After insilico analysis, several differentially expressed miRNAs were found to be the regulators of genes linked with inflammation and play paramount roles in the development of DNP. Thus, their results point towards the contribution of abrupt levels of miRNAs to the pathogenesis of DNP [73].

Literature supports that expression levels of miRNA also depends upon the type of traumatic injury. For example, axotomy up regulates the expression of miR-1 whereas ligation of the sciatic nerve down regulates its expression in DRG. Likewise, ligation of the sciatic nerve down regulates the expression of miR-206 in the DRG but axotomy does not [65]. Another observation seen in animal models is that nerve damage may be functionally recovered by alterations in miRNA expression. For example, after nerve injury, increased levels of miR-21 were found to be implicated in neuropathic pain and axon growth [67, 74]. Similarly, neurite outgrowth was reported after up regulation of miR-222 following sciatic nerve transection [75]. In addition, nerve injury in mice induced miR-431 expression which in turn repressed the antagonist of Wnt/beta-catenin signaling *i.e.* Kremen1 and thus triggered regenerative axon growth [76]. As all these studies show dramatic changes in expression levels of miRNAs in broad variety of animal models of pain, pointing miRNAs as fundamental regulators of pain pathophysiology. Hence, by enlightening and elucidating the signaling pathways modulated by common miRNAs which got altered in most of the animal models would add new dimension to our understanding of the pathophysiology of pain.

Regulation of MicroRNAs in Peripheral Somatic Sensory Neurons

Any noxious stimuli (such as heat, cold, pressure or acid) or inflammation is first sensed by peripheral sensory neurons whose soma lie in the DRG or TG and their axon terminals innervate the skin and other organs and then they transduce this physicochemical stimulus into an electrochemical one by causing changes in neuronal membrane potentials and then transmit this nociceptive information to the spinal and medullary dorsal horns respectively [5, 6]. Researchers have employed several preclinical neuropathic models of mouse and rat species including sciatic nerve injury, chronic constriction injury (CCI) and spinal nerve ligation (SNL) to study miRNA biology in neuropathic pain states. MiRNA deregulation is not only studied in neuropathic pain but has also been studied in mouse models of inflammatory pain [*e.g.*, involving peripheral hind-paw inflammation with Freund's Complete Adjuvant (CFA) or carrageenan] and even models of early hypersensitivity evoked by peripheral formalin injection [2, 4]. Cancer of any tissue is also a cause of chronic pain and it is mediated *via* the peripheral and central mechanisms. Only one report claimed to study miRNA profile in tumor mediated pain conditions where authors observed dysregulation of 57 miRNAs in the DRG of a bone metastasis pain model as compared to tumor affected areas (Table **1**). The study further revealed that these miRNAs were involved in the maintenance and not in the development phase of tumor-mediated hyperalgesia. The authors observed that miR-1a-3p, miR-34c-5p, and miR-370-3p were found to have pro-nociceptive effects. Up regulation of miR-1a-3p has been reported in the DRG in bone metastatic pain model and the tumor-associated pain was obliterated by the treatment of miR-1a-3p inhibitor. Gene Clcn3 which is a chloride channel was found to be a direct target of miR-1a-3p which then modulated the pain perception (Table **2**) [69]. Further research is warranted in miRNA mediating cancer associated pain to gain more depth of regulatory networks of miRNA and target genes in cancer pain. In harmony, by regulating neuronal excitability, miR-7a was shown to play a significant role in maintaining the late phase of neuropathic pain while in contrast, over expression of the same miRNA did not affect the inflammatory or other physiological pain. This could be explained by the observation that during inflammatory pain, there occur no changes in expression of miR-7a [68]. MiR-7a has been found to target the β2 subunit of voltage-gated sodium channels and thus, expression of these channels on cell surface is affected which increases neuronal excitability (Table **2**) [77]. A cluster of miRNA which is consistently down regulated in different pain models is miR-182-96-183 cluster. This cluster is made up of three different miRNAs *i.e.* miR-182, miR-96 and miR-183 which found their location on an intergenic region of human chromosome 7q and transcribed as polycistronic miRNA. Expression of this cluster has been observed to be specific to sensory organs and is found to be down regulated in ipsilateral DRGs in several neuropathic, inflammatory pain models and osteoarthritic pain [78 - 80]. CFA injection cause the down regulation of miR-183 within a few hours in TG into the rat masseter muscle during inflammatory muscle pain (Table **1**) [81]. The miRNAs of this cluster target key ion channels (Table **2**) and thus modulate pain transmission, hence cellular interference of this cluster may have concerted impact on pain modulation. In sheer contrast, is miR-21 whose expression is up regulated in DRG neurons during several nerve injuries [67, 68, 74, 82, 83] and surprisingly, during neuropathic pain induction by interleukin (IL)-1b injection in rats, levels of miR-21 were found to be increased in intact rats [68]. It was further involved in the maintenance of neuropathic pain (Table **1**) [67]. Several targets of miR-21 related to pain pathways have been validated and shown to modulate the neuropathic pain (Table **2**).

Table 2. list of validated targets of differentially regulated miRNAs in different pain models

miRNA	Validated Target	Pain condition/Model	Reference
DRG			
miR-1a-3p	Chloride channel 3	Cancer pain	[2]
miR-7a	Sodium channel, voltage-gated, type II, beta; Nav1.2	Neuropathic pain	[131]
miR-96	Sodium channel, voltage – gated, type III, alpha Nav1.3	Neuropathic pain	[74]
Antisense – Kcna2	Potassium voltage – gated channel subfamily A member 2	Neuropathic pain	[132]
miR -183	Sodium channel, voltage – gated, type III, alpha Nav1.3	Neuropathic pain	[78]
miR - 134	M – opioid receptor, mOR	Inflammatory pain	[126]
miR-1a-3p	Chloride Channel 3	Bone cancer CFA	[65, 69]
miR-34c-5p	Unknown	Bone cancer	[69]
miR-183	$Na_v1.3$, BDNF	SNL	[82]
miR-182-96-183 cluster	BDNF, Substance P, Voltage-dependent sodium channels (NaV1.3 and NaV1.7), Voltage-dependent calcium channel subunit $\alpha2\delta1$	Inflammatory muscle pain, Neuropathic pain	[79, 81]

(Table 2) contd.....

miRNA	Validated Target	Pain condition/Model	Reference
miR-21	Negative regulators of matrix metalloproteinases (Reck and timp-3), extracellular signal-regulated kinase (sprout 1, sprout 2 and Btg2), Endogenous inhibitor of phosphatidylinositol 3-kinase	Neuropathic pain	[133 - 135]
TG			
miR-124a	MeCP2	Formalin (Dorsal Spinal)	[2]
Spinal Dorsal Horn			
miR - 103	Cav1.2–comprising L-type calcium channel	Neuropathic pain	[115]
miR - 124	Methyl CpG-binding protein 2	Inflammatory pain	[70]
miR-23b	NADPH oxidase 4	SCI	[129]
miR-195	ATG14	SNL	[130]
Brain			
miR-200b and miR-429	DNA-methyltransferase 3a	Neuropathic pain	[136]
miR-155	CCAAT/enhancer binding protein Beta	Inflammatory pain	[96]
miR-let-7a,c,g	μ opioid receptor	Opioid tolerance (Brain)	[98]

Different studies till now highlighted different deregulated miRNAs among different pain models, making it a difficult task to find common miRNAs for pain modulation from therapy point of view. For example, during neuropathic pain induction, miRNAs such as miR-34 family members, miR-33a, miR-369-5p, miR-142-5p and miR-218 were strongly down regulated [84], however, they were strongly up regulated following bone metastatic pain induction in ipsilateral DRGs (Table **1**) [69]. There is sheer contrast in the regulation of a few miRNAs across different models of neuropathic pain itself. For instance, decreased levels of miR-1 were observed in DRG on partial nerve injury where its inconsistent increased levels have been detected in a sciatic nerve axotomy (SNA) model [65]. Therefore, these miRNA profiling results are subject to provide sheer variations in the knowledge of miRNA biology in nociceptive modulation and therefore, should be interpreted carefully keeping in mind all the parameters of the experiments including method, platform and time point.

Regulation of MiRNAs in the Spinal Cord

Spinal cord is made up of dorsal and ventral horn. Spinal cord dorsal horn (SDH) is the place for secondary neurons where processing and integration of the information provided by primary sensory neurons occur and which then transmit the signals to the brain for further action. Interestingly, any abnormal transformation of sensory information at the spinal cord level plays a dominant role in the initiation and maintenance of chronic pain from both spinal and peripheral origins. As several studies reported deregulation of miRNAs in neuropathic pain, therefore, analyzing miRNA expression and miRNA mediated signaling pathways in the SDH in different pain models may help in highlighting molecular mechanisms underlying pain. During the miRNA profiling using TaqMan array technology in chronic constriction injury (CCI) rat model, differential expression of several miRNAs was reported in the dorsal spinal cord as compared to their sham groups. Some of them including miR-21, -500 and -221 were found to be related to neuropathic pain [85]. Further, Brandenburger *et al.* reported up regulation of miRNAs-494, -720, -690 and -668 in the same model of neuropathic pain in rats. However, induction of neuropathic pain by CCI did not induce marked changes in the expression of highly expressed miRNAs *i.e.* miR-124 and let-7 family in the spinal cord at any studied time point (Table **1**) [86]. Several reports documented a decrease in the expressions of a plethora of miRNAs including miR-203, -103, -1, -124, -129-1, 129-1, -124a, -146a during various days in SDH in different models of neuropathic pain in rat and mice (Table **1**) [74, 87 - 92]. Interestingly, several common miRNAs showed similar expression patterns in pain states in both the spinal cord as well as in the DRG [5]. For instance, induction of osteoarthritic pain caused marked reduction in the levels of miR-182-96-183 cluster and miR-146a in DRG as well as spinal cord [80]. Similarly, during induction of inflammatory and neuropathic pain, differential expression of miR-1, miR-16 and miR-206 was observed in both the DRG and dorsal spinal cord (Table **1**) [65]. Although expression profile of a plethora of miRNAs in spinal cord is available yet scanty information is there about the miRNA functions in the processing of spinal pain during chronic pain states.

Expression of MiRNAs in other Brain Regions involved in Pain

As the final action has to be taken by brain after all processing and transmission of information to the brain, hence it is of paramount importance to look for the miRNA profile of the areas of brain which are potentially involved in pain modulations. Besides this, it is hypothesized that high order brain functions including anxiety, cognitive and mood can be affected by chronic pain by altering the miRNA profiles of brain areas involved in these functions. Although the specific contributions of diverse brain regions and circuits in pain remain unclear, yet research has been put forward in pieces to reveal the biological functions of miRNAs in brain with respect to pain pathophysiology. In hippocampus, miR-132 and miR-125b were differentially expressed during neuropathic and inflammatory pain conditions (Table **1**) [93, 94]. Surprisingly, neuropathic and inflammatory pain conditions evoked marked modulations of common miRNAs in the hippocampus which suggests that at the higher order of central nervous system, common miRNA dysregulation is caused by chronic pain irrespective of the causes of pain, which is complete contrast to the case for the spinal cord and DRG [5]. In the nucleus accumbens, which plays a major role in reward circuit, levels of miR-200b and miR-429 were decreased during neuropathic pain state after partial sciatic nerve ligation but not in hippocampus, frontal cortex or amygdala (Table **1**) [95]. Further, miRNA expression profile was determined in the prefrontal cortex by Poh *et al.*, which suggests increased activity concurrent with altered nociceptive thresholds in animal models [96]. In carrageenan-induced facial inflammatory pain mouse model, expression levels of miR-223 and miR-155 were found to be increased (Table **1**) [97]. Similarly, after morphine treatment, up regulation of the let-7 family members was detected in the brain and this family modulated opioid antinociceptive tolerance by targeting the μ opioid receptor (Table **2**) [98].

Extracellular MiRNA can Function as Neuromodulator

As discussed above, alterations have been observed in the expression of substantial number of miRNAs in somatosensory system during chronic pain. Recently, Ru-Rong Ji's group has provided a new dimension to the miRNA study in pain pathology. They showed that extracellular application of miR-let-7b induced rapid voltage dependent inward ionic currents as well as action potentials in DRG neurons. Here, Let-7b behaved as an extracellular ligand and got bound to toll-like receptor-7 (TLR7)/TRPA1 ion channel. After sequence specific binding, let-7b induced TLR7/TRPA1-dependent single channel activities in HEK293 cells over-expressing TLR7/TRPA1 as well as DRG neurons. Further, let-7b elicited rapid spontaneous pain following intraplantar injection *via* TLR7 and TRPA1 [99]. They also observed release of let-7b in the extracellular medium from DRG neurons after neuronal activation by capsaicin or depolarization with potassium chloride, which suggests that this miRNA could either function on nociceptors in an autocrine manner or may lead to a novel regulatory signaling. Formalin-induced TRPA1 currents and spontaneous pain was reduced by the application of let-7b inhibitor. Thus, they suggested that by activating TLR7/TRPA1 in nociceptive neurons, these secreted extracellular miRNAs may serve as novel pain modulators. They also hypothesized a debut neurotransmitter like function of Let-7b [99]. Genome wide changes in the miRNA secreting cells can be reflected by these extracellular miRNAs [5]. Previous studies have also detected extracellular miRNAs in various disease states, including pain. A report suggested a link between the levels of many miRNAs in blood with the symptoms of complex regional pain syndrome in affected people [100]. Thus, from these studies one can imagine that time is not far when levels of extracellular miRNAs will provide the information about the chronic pain.

Translational aspect of MiRNA Biology in Pain Therapeutics

Research over the last few years has implicated miRNA alterations in the patho-mechanisms of pain which may have triggered the establishment of various diseases/disorders associated with chronic pain. The vigorous changes in expression and functions of miRNAs in different pain pathways have confronted the major obstacles before incorporating miRNA based pharmacological interventions into treatment of pain [24]. Recent technology has developed various tools to either enhance the expression of a particular miRNA or dampen its expression. The instrumental role of miRNAs in different pain conditions combined with the remarkable stability of extracellular miRNAs raises the possibility of development of miRNA-targeted therapies for the pain related diseases / disorders caused by their deregulation.

Prediction and Experimental Validation of MiRNA Targets

MicroRNAs perform their function against a specific phenotype by regulating the expression of their target mRNAs inside the cells. They modulate gene expression either by repression of translation or by degradation of the target message or both (Fig. **1**) [25, 101]. Hence, elucidating molecular mechanisms underlying miRNA action includes the identification and function of the genes which are specifically targets of individual miRNAs. Prediction of animal miRNA targets has been a daunting task because pairing between miRNAs with their targets includes just 2-9 nucleotides. For the prediction of targets of miRNAs, a handful of computational algorithms have been developed till now which are not free of several demerits [102 - 104]. Although these algorithms have used several parameters to predict the miRNA-mRNA interactions and provide thousands of targets for a single miRNA, yet functional evaluation of these thousands of miRNA-mRNA pairs becomes impossible. Hence, to improve the accuracy of binding site prediction, one can increase the stringency of miRNA target prediction and employ several algorithms simultaneously and can choose the common targets between several algorithms. This will enhance the chance of the selected target to be a valid one. Another approach is to employ a system level analysis to identify the function to be modulated by the miRNA [6]. Another approach that can directly validate miRNA-mRNA target pair is to perform the expression analysis for the predicted targets after the treatment of cells with miRNA expression modulators. Functional interaction between miRNA-mRNA target pair can be validated using reporter experiments after the selection of a single or numerous target genes for a single miRNA (reviewed in [105]). These reporter constructs harbor miRNA binding site of the target gene under the control of a reporter promoter and the effect of miRNA of interest can be directly assessed in *in vitro* system. Further, with the help of miRNA mimics and inhibitors, the expression of their targets can be assessed both at RNA and protein levels. Thus, validation of miRNA targets will help in elucidating the molecular mechanism underlying miRNA function.

Tools to Upregulate MiRNA for Replacement Therapies

Intracellular miRNAs can be up regulated by miRNA mimics in an efficient way.

MiRNA mimics are double-stranded RNA molecules that harbor the exact sequence of endogenous miRNAs and behave like the latter upon cellular uptake. As this is a double stranded structure, hence the strand which harbors the targeted mature miRNA sequence is named as the 'active strand' or 'guide strand' whereas the second strand becomes the 'inactive strand' or 'passive strand'. The active strand gets preferentially incorporated into the RISC, whereas the passive strand gets degraded (Fig. **1**) [6]. Several proprietary chemical modifications have been applied to promote preferential integration as well as stability of the guide strand into the RISC. Passive strand can be conjugated with cholesterol to facilitate cellular uptake whereas active strand can be conjugated with fluorescein isothiocyanate (FITC) to facilitate localization following uptake in peripheral sensory neurons [69]. This technique has already made its way to clinical trials. For example, the first miRNA replacement compound that has reached phase I clinical trials is MRX34 which mimics miR-34a. Some of the patients suffering from primary liver cancer or metastatic cancer of liver received intravenous delivery of miR-34 mimic conjugated with liposome (http://clinicaltrials.gov/ct2/show/NCT01829971).

<u>Tools for Antagonizing or Attenuating MiRNAs for Inhibitory Therapy</u>

The nuisance miRNAs which drive disease initiation and/or progression can be blocked by specific miRNA inhibitors. Chemical modifications are also available for these inhibitors to make them stable and highly efficient. For example, anti-miRNA oligonucleotides (AMOs) which are chemically modified have been developed long back to inhibit endogenous miRNA expression. Either whole miRNA sequence or the seed sequence of the mature miRNA can be targeted by these AMOs [6, 106, 107]. They contain proprietary modifications to individual nucleotides (such as 2' Fluoro, 2',4'-methylene, 2'-O-methoxyethyl, 2'-O-methyl, morpholino and Locked nucleic acid) or modifications to the backbone (such as phosphorothioate linkage) which have their own advantages. Locked nucleic acid (LNA) is a bicyclic RNA analogue in which the ribose moiety is modified by the formation of a 2'-O,4'-C methylene bridge. Modifications are incorporated at the 2' position of the ribose moiety in the 2'-fluoro (2'-F), 2'-O-methyl (2'-O-Me) and 2'-O-methoxyethyl (2'-MOE) nucleotides, whereas in case of morpholino oligomers, the sugar moiety is replaced by a six-membered morpholine ring.

However, in the phosphorothioate (PS) linkage, one of the non-bridging oxygen atoms is replaced by sulfur in the phosphate group [108]. Thus, depending upon the manufacturer, chemistry and conjugations employed, AMOs are known by different names, such as 'antagomirs', 'antimiRs' and 'miRNA inhibitors' [109, 110]. After their entry into the cells, AMOs bind to and sequester the targeted miRNA and thus make the specific miRNA unavailable for RISC incorporation and in this way, increase the expression of their targets (Fig. **1**). Antagomir constitutes another category of anti-miRNA sequences which are conjugated with cholesterol and have been exploited for the inhibition of specific miRNA expression in brain regions following intra cerebroventricular (i.c.v.) delivery [111]. However, they were highly inefficient in inhibiting targeted miRNA in DRGs following intrathecal (i.t.) delivery [69]. Another category includes LNA-based miRNA inhibitors which have been widely employed and resulted in increased cellular uptake into DRGs following i.t. delivery [69]. Although technology is available to down regulate the expression of miRNA in a particular pain condition and thus can provide relieve from different types of pains yet delivery of AMO and breaching into the nervous system *in vivo* and efficacy are major obstacle in the path of development of miRNA based pain therapeutics.

However, recent studies have used the technology to a far new limit and created hope for miRNA based drugs. For instance, Miravirsen which is an LNA-antagomir against miR-122 has successfully gone through two phases: phase I clinical trials and a phase IIa clinical trial against human hepatitis C virus infection [112]. Another antisense technology developed for the inhibition of miR-33 uses 2′-fluoro-methoxyethyl-phosphorothioate chemistry and has been efficiently administered into African Green monkeys subcutaneously for elucidating the therapeutic cure of cardiovascular diseases [113].

Other Novel Approaches to Alter MiRNA Expression

Researchers have employed several novel approaches to modulate miRNA expression *in vivo*. Several viruses including adenoviruses, lentiviruses and herpes simplex viruses have been engineered to encode either specific miRNA inhibiting sequences or precursor miRNA sequences. Virions, the infectious particle designed for transmission of genetic material among hosts, have been successfully delivered into the SDH or DRG by i.t. means for the knock down of specific genes. The advantage of these virions is that single injection of either miRNA inhibitor or precursor miRNA is sufficient to show effects over long time [114, 115]. Besides specific single miRNA inhibition, microRNA sponges have been discovered by Ebert *et al.* which can be used to inhibit individual miRNAs or a family of miRNAs. These miRNA sponges are the competitive inhibitors/transcripts which usually require strong promoters for their expression and contain multiple, tandem binding sites for microRNA of interest or a family of miRNAs. These sponges are usually encoded by vectors and upon their transient transfections into cell culture system; they suppress miRNAs and derepress their targets as efficiently as other chemically modified inhibitors [116]. Another efficient approach to study miRNA's function is to generate transgenic knockout mice which lack miRNA processing enzymes Dicer, Drosha, DGCR8 and Ago2. Absence of miRNA manufacturing machinery will lead to the global loss of microRNAs and render the transgenic mice embryonically lethal [117]. However, knockout mice with specific deletion of Dicer in sensory neurons have been generated [70]. Deletion of Dicer will result in the abrogation of all miRNAs, hence over expression or knock down studies can be performed in these transgenic mice. However, knowledge regarding intricate circuits involving other miRNAs in action with miRNA of interest and biological function of individual miRNA will be restricted. Besides this, embryonic stem (ES) cell repositories carrying knock out of most of known mouse miRNA genes are also available and these cells can be exploited to generate specific knockout allelic lines to reveal the functions of miRNA of interest [118]. Another technology which is paving its way to provide solutions to the miRNA therapeutics is nanoparticle technology. Inorganic nanoparticles including silicon oxide, gold and calcium phosphate have already been used for the efficient delivery of miRNA mimics or inhibitors into different cellular systems *in vitro* [119, 120] as well as *in vivo via* systemic delivery [121, 122]. Any of these techniques can be adopted for the successful delivery of miRNA modulators in a sensory neuron specific manner to study the effect of miRNA of interest.

Roadblocks in Translating MiRNA Biology to Pain Therapeutics

Based on the distinct modulations in miRNA expression during specific pain state, the scientific society can have high spirit that these small non-coding RNAs can either serve as biomarkers of specific pain states or can be intervened as therapeutic targets. Besides the significant advantages of miRNAs in being small in size, known sequence, evolutionary conservation and benefits from antisense technologies yet there are several road blocks which need to be clear before incorporation of miRNA research into clinical trials. One of the biggest challenges in pain research in nervous system is of specific delivery of miRNA inhibitors and/or mimics into the target tissue particularly in the SDH and DRG. Literature suggest that various approaches have been employed to deliver miRNA inhibitors or mimics into neuronal tissue, such as direct injection into the brain/spinal cord parenchyma or delivery to the corresponding compartments of the cerebrospinal fluid *via* i.c.v. or i.t. injection [6]. MiRNA inhibitors together with a chemical reagent to modulate specific miRNA expression have been delivered in the SDH or DRG to investigate the phenotypic effects of over expression or loss of function of miRNA on pain [69, 91]. Recently, it has been shown that intravenous delivery of miRNA inhibitors and mimics modulated their expression in SDH neurons [2]. This is more acceptable from the clinical point of view, but this is more prone to wide-scale side effects often seen at the systemic level. Another lacuna of intravenous administration is that sufficient amounts of miRNA modulators do not get delivered into sensory neurons of somato-sensory system although Alvarez-Erviti *et al.* claims to deliver a siRNA by systemic injection of exosomes to oligodendrocytes, microglia and neurons by breaching blood brain barrier in mouse [123]. Currently, miRNA-based therapy is not available as oral formulations which is the most preferable way and is well-tolerated in most patients [5]. These are some of the obstacles associated with the future of miRNA therapeutics for pain management that need to be crossed before their clinical use.

CONCLUDING REMARKS AND FUTURE PERSPECTIVES

Chronic pain is such a debilitating condition that can emerge into various pain disorders including cystitis-induced chronic pain, irritable bowel disorder and complex regional pain syndrome if remain unmanaged. Several pioneering studies have advanced our knowledge of various different roles of miRNAs in chronic pain. Substantial changes in the miRNA expression profile occur during several pain conditions in almost every component of somato sensory system from peripheral primary neurons to higher central nervous system neurons. It has also revealed by literature that miRNAs play decent functional roles in the modulation of pain perception and they have been selected as promising therapeutic targets for therapeutic intervention of chronic pain. However, molecular mechanism underlying changes in their expression during different pain conditions remains elusive due to the experimental validation of a very few target genes of these miRNAs. Because the biological effect of a miRNA depends upon the functions of its targets, hence it is of utmost interest to increase the efficiency of validation of miRNA target pair using unbiased approaches including miRNA sensors, decoy libraries and high-throughput sequencing of RNA isolated by cross linking immunoprecipitation (HITS-CLIP), PAR-CLIP and TAP-Tar. Also, our understanding of transcriptional modulation of miRNAs in pain is hampered due to restricted knowledge of the promoter regions and transcription start sites of these miRNAs. MiRNAs have tremendous potential to regulate a plethora of targets and hence multiple signaling pathways simultaneously and recently, they have been described as intercellular communicator. Hence, care should be taken during the intravenous delivery of these miRNAs in pain models as they can evoke genome wide changes in neighboring cells beside targeted one. Therefore, it is of utmost importance to further advance our understanding about the mechanism of action of miRNAs in pain modulations which can simultaneously advance the field of antisense chemistry, *in vivo* delivery, miRNA efficacy and stability. Addressing these research areas will set a milestone for the use of miRNA in the generation of analgesics for the pain treatment. Future investigations are warranted in exploring the target genes of miRNAs from pain perception to modulation that will further advance our understanding of the pleiotropic functions of miRNA and complexity of the gene regulatory networks required for the pain modulation. Thus, miRNA research can provide new dimensions to both basic biology of pain and translational medicine in near future.

CONFLICT OF INTEREST

The authors confirm that they have no conflict of interest to declare for this publication.

ACKNOWLEDGEMENTS

We acknowledge Tanya and Karnika for their help. We thank Prof. Subrata Sinha, Director, NBRC for the kind support. This work was supported by the INSPIRE Faculty fellowship awarded to Y.K.A (Code-IFA 13-LSBM-90) by the Department of Science and Technology (DST) and Indian National Science Academy (INSA) and National Brain Research Centre (NBRC) core funds, Manesar, India. The funding agency had no role in the writing of the chapter or in the decision to submit this chapter for publication.

ABBREVIATIONS

DRG	Dorsal root ganglion
HITS CLIP	High-throughput sequencing of RNA isolated by crosslinking immunoprecipitation
MicroRNA	miRNA
PAR-CLIP	Photoactivatable-ribonucleoside-enhanced crosslinking and immunoprecipitation
TG	Trigeminal ganglion
TAP-Tar	Tandem affinity purification of miRNA target mRNAs

REFERENCES

[1] Andersen HH, Duroux M, Gazerani P. MicroRNAs as modulators and biomarkers of inflammatory and neuropathic pain conditions. Neurobiol Dis 2014; 71: 159-68. [http://dx.doi.org/10.1016/j.nbd.2014.08.003] [PMID: 25119878]

[2] Kynast KL, Russe OQ, Geisslinger G, Niederberger E. Novel findings in pain processing pathways: implications for miRNAs as future therapeutic targets. Expert Rev Neurother 2013; 13(5): 515-25. [http://dx.doi.org/10.1586/ern.13.34] [PMID: 23621309]

[3] Lutz BM, Bekker A, Tao YX. Noncoding RNAs: new players in chronic pain. Anesthesiology 2014; 121(2): 409-17. [http://dx.doi.org/10.1097/ALN.0000000000000265] [PMID: 24739997]

[4] Niederberger E, Kynast K, Lötsch J, Geisslinger G. MicroRNAs as new players in the pain game. Pain 2011; 152(7): 1455-8. [http://dx.doi.org/10.1016/j.pain.2011.01.042] [PMID: 21353390]

[5] Sakai A, Suzuki H. Emerging roles of microRNAs in chronic pain. Neurochem Int 2014; 77: 58-67. [http://dx.doi.org/10.1016/j.neuint.2014.05.010] [PMID: 24905749]

[6] Bali KK, Kuner R. Noncoding RNAs: key molecules in understanding and treating pain. Trends Mol Med 2014; 20(8): 437-48. [http://dx.doi.org/10.1016/j.molmed.2014.05.006] [PMID: 24986063]

[7] Dworkin RH, O'Connor AB, Kent J, *et al.* Interventional management of neuropathic pain: NeuPSIG recommendations. Pain 2013; 154(11): 2249-61.
[http://dx.doi.org/10.1016/j.pain.2013.06.004] [PMID: 23748119]

[8] Kuner R. Central mechanisms of pathological pain. Nat Med 2010; 16(11): 1258-66.
[http://dx.doi.org/10.1038/nm.2231] [PMID: 20948531]

[9] Todd AJ. Neuronal circuitry for pain processing in the dorsal horn. Nature reviews 2010; 11: 823-36.
[http://dx.doi.org/10.1038/nrn2947]

[10] Apkarian AV. The brain in chronic pain: clinical implications. Pain Manag 2011; 1(6): 577-86.
[http://dx.doi.org/10.2217/pmt.11.53] [PMID: 22140414]

[11] McWilliams LA, Cox BJ, Enns MW. Mood and anxiety disorders associated with chronic pain: an examination in a nationally representative sample. Pain 2003; 106(1-2): 127-33.
[http://dx.doi.org/10.1016/S0304-3959(03)00301-4] [PMID: 14581119]

[12] Jones-Rhoades MW, Bartel DP, Bartel B. MicroRNAS and their regulatory roles in plants. Annu Rev Plant Biol 2006; 57: 19-53.
[http://dx.doi.org/10.1146/annurev.arplant.57.032905.105218] [PMID: 16669754]

[13] Grimson A, Srivastava M, Fahey B, *et al.* Early origins and evolution of microRNAs and Piwi-interacting RNAs in animals. Nature 2008; 455(7217): 1193-7.
[http://dx.doi.org/10.1038/nature07415] [PMID: 18830242]

[14] Lee RC, Feinbaum RL, Ambros V. The C. elegans heterochronic gene lin-4 encodes small RNAs with antisense complementarity to lin-14. Cell 1993; 75(5): 843-54.
[http://dx.doi.org/10.1016/0092-8674(93)90529-Y] [PMID: 8252621]

[15] Wightman B, Ha I, Ruvkun G. Posttranscriptional regulation of the heterochronic gene lin-14 by lin-4 mediates temporal pattern formation in C. elegans. Cell 1993; 75(5): 855-62.
[http://dx.doi.org/10.1016/0092-8674(93)90530-4] [PMID: 8252622]

[16] Slack FJ, Basson M, Liu Z, Ambros V, Horvitz HR, Ruvkun G. The lin-41 RBCC gene acts in the C. elegans heterochronic pathway between the let-7 regulatory RNA and the LIN-29 transcription factor. Mol Cell 2000; 5(4): 659-69.
[http://dx.doi.org/10.1016/S1097-2765(00)80245-2] [PMID: 10882102]

[17] Karp X, Ambros V. Encountering microRNAs in cell fate signaling. Science. Developmental biology 2005; 310: 1288-9.

[18] Chen CZ, *et al.* MicroRNAs modulate hematopoietic lineage differentiation 2004.
[http://dx.doi.org/10.1126/science.1091903]

[19] Stadler BM, Ruohola-Baker H. Small RNAs: keeping stem cells in line. Cell 2008; 132(4): 563-6.
[http://dx.doi.org/10.1016/j.cell.2008.02.005] [PMID: 18295575]

[20] Yi R, Poy MN, Stoffel M, Fuchs E. A skin microRNA promotes differentiation by repressing 'stemness'. Nature 2008; 452(7184): 225-9.
[http://dx.doi.org/10.1038/nature06642] [PMID: 18311128]

[21] Lynam-Lennon N, Maher SG, Reynolds JV. The roles of microRNA in cancer and apoptosis. Biol Rev Camb Philos Soc 2009; 84(1): 55-71.

[http://dx.doi.org/10.1111/j.1469-185X.2008.00061.x] [PMID: 19046400]

[22] Leung AK, Sharp PA. MicroRNA functions in stress responses. Mol Cell 2010; 40(2): 205-15. [http://dx.doi.org/10.1016/j.molcel.2010.09.027] [PMID: 20965416]

[23] Rottiers V, Näär AM. MicroRNAs in metabolism and metabolic disorders. Nat Rev Mol Cell Biol 2012; 13(4): 239-50. [http://dx.doi.org/10.1038/nrm3313] [PMID: 22436747]

[24] Quiat D, Olson EN. MicroRNAs in cardiovascular disease: from pathogenesis to prevention and treatment. J Clin Invest 2013; 123(1): 11-8. [http://dx.doi.org/10.1172/JCI62876] [PMID: 23281405]

[25] Adlakha YK, Saini N. Brain microRNAs and insights into biological functions and therapeutic potential of brain enriched miRNA-128. Mol Cancer 2014; 13: 33. [http://dx.doi.org/10.1186/1476-4598-13-33] [PMID: 24555688]

[26] Di Leva G, Garofalo M, Croce CM. MicroRNAs in cancer. Annu Rev Pathol 2014; 9: 287-314. [http://dx.doi.org/10.1146/annurev-pathol-012513-104715] [PMID: 24079833]

[27] Abe M, Bonini NM. MicroRNAs and neurodegeneration: role and impact. Trends Cell Biol 2013; 23(1): 30-6. [http://dx.doi.org/10.1016/j.tcb.2012.08.013] [PMID: 23026030]

[28] Chen H, Lan HY, Roukos DH, Cho WC. Application of microRNAs in diabetes mellitus. J Endocrinol 2014; 222(1): R1-R10. [http://dx.doi.org/10.1530/JOE-13-0544] [PMID: 24781254]

[29] Swaminathan S, Murray DD, Kelleher AD. The role of microRNAs in HIV-1 pathogenesis and therapy. AIDS 2012; 26(11): 1325-34. [http://dx.doi.org/10.1097/QAD.0b013e328352adca] [PMID: 22382145]

[30] Shrivastava S, Steele R, Ray R, Ray RB. MicroRNAs: Role in Hepatitis C Virus pathogenesis. Genes Dis 2015; 2(1): 35-45. [http://dx.doi.org/10.1016/j.gendis.2015.01.001] [PMID: 25984557]

[31] Bhalala OG, Srikanth M, Kessler JA. The emerging roles of microRNAs in CNS injuries. Nat Rev Neurol 2013; 9(6): 328-39. [http://dx.doi.org/10.1038/nrneurol.2013.67] [PMID: 23588363]

[32] Bartel DP. MicroRNAs: target recognition and regulatory functions. Cell 2009; 136(2): 215-33. [http://dx.doi.org/10.1016/j.cell.2009.01.002] [PMID: 19167326]

[33] Lagos-Quintana M, *et al.* Identification of novel genes coding for small expressed RNAs. Science 2001; 294: 853-8. [http://dx.doi.org/10.1126/science.1064921]

[34] Ørom UA, Nielsen FC, Lund AH. MicroRNA-10a binds the 5'UTR of ribosomal protein mRNAs and enhances their translation. Mol Cell 2008; 30(4): 460-71. [http://dx.doi.org/10.1016/j.molcel.2008.05.001] [PMID: 18498749]

[35] Henke JI, Goergen D, Zheng J, *et al.* microRNA-122 stimulates translation of hepatitis C virus RNA. EMBO J 2008; 27(24): 3300-10. [http://dx.doi.org/10.1038/emboj.2008.244] [PMID: 19020517]

[36] Tay Y, Zhang J, Thomson AM, Lim B, Rigoutsos I. MicroRNAs to Nanog, Oct4 and Sox2 coding regions modulate embryonic stem cell differentiation. Nature 2008; 455(7216): 1124-8. [http://dx.doi.org/10.1038/nature07299] [PMID: 18806776]

[37] Huang S, Wu S, Ding J, *et al.* MicroRNA-181a modulates gene expression of zinc finger family members by directly targeting their coding regions. Nucleic Acids Res 2010; 38(20): 7211-8. [http://dx.doi.org/10.1093/nar/gkq564] [PMID: 20591824]

[38] Duursma AM, *et al.* miR-148 targets human DNMT3b protein coding region. RNA, New York, NY 2008; 14: 872-7.

[39] Rogers K, Chen X. Biogenesis, turnover, and mode of action of plant microRNAs. Plant Cell 2013; 25(7): 2383-99. [http://dx.doi.org/10.1105/tpc.113.113159] [PMID: 23881412]

[40] Pillai RS, Bhattacharyya SN, Filipowicz W. Repression of protein synthesis by miRNAs: how many mechanisms? Trends Cell Biol 2007; 17(3): 118-26. [http://dx.doi.org/10.1016/j.tcb.2006.12.007] [PMID: 17197185]

[41] Wu W, Sun M, Zou GM, Chen J. MicroRNA and cancer: Current status and prospective. Int J Cancer 2007; 120(5): 953-60. [http://dx.doi.org/10.1002/ijc.22454] [PMID: 17163415]

[42] Peterson KJ, Dietrich MR, McPeek MA. MicroRNAs and metazoan macroevolution: insights into canalization, complexity, and the Cambrian explosion. BioEssays 2009; 31(7): 736-47. [http://dx.doi.org/10.1002/bies.200900033] [PMID: 19472371]

[43] Rodriguez A, Griffiths-Jones S, Ashurst JL, Bradley A. Identification of mammalian microRNA host genes and transcription units. Genome Res 2004; 14(10A): 1902-10. [http://dx.doi.org/10.1101/gr.2722704] [PMID: 15364901]

[44] Griffiths-Jones S. Annotating noncoding RNA genes. Annu Rev Genomics Hum Genet 2007; 8: 279-98. [http://dx.doi.org/10.1146/annurev.genom.8.080706.092419] [PMID: 17506659]

[45] Ul Hussain M. Micro-RNAs (miRNAs): genomic organisation, biogenesis and mode of action. Cell Tissue Res 2012; 349(2): 405-13. [http://dx.doi.org/10.1007/s00441-012-1438-0] [PMID: 22622804]

[46] Lee Y, Ahn C, Han J, *et al.* The nuclear RNase III Drosha initiates microRNA processing. Nature 2003; 425(6956): 415-9. [http://dx.doi.org/10.1038/nature01957] [PMID: 14508493]

[47] Han J, Lee Y, Yeom KH, Kim YK, Jin H, Kim VN. The Drosha-DGCR8 complex in primary microRNA processing. Genes Dev 2004; 18(24): 3016-27. [http://dx.doi.org/10.1101/gad.1262504] [PMID: 15574589]

[48] Gregory RI, Yan KP, Amuthan G, *et al.* The Microprocessor complex mediates the genesis of microRNAs. Nature 2004; 432(7014): 235-40. [http://dx.doi.org/10.1038/nature03120] [PMID: 15531877]

[49] Kim YK, Kim VN. Processing of intronic microRNAs. EMBO J 2007; 26(3): 775-83. [http://dx.doi.org/10.1038/sj.emboj.7601512] [PMID: 17255951]

[50] Okamura K, Hagen JW, Duan H, Tyler DM, Lai EC. The mirtron pathway generates microRNA-class regulatory RNAs in Drosophila. Cell 2007; 130(1): 89-100.
[http://dx.doi.org/10.1016/j.cell.2007.06.028] [PMID: 17599402]

[51] Lund E, *et al.* Nuclear export of microRNA precursors. Science 2004; 303: 95-8.
[http://dx.doi.org/10.1126/science.1090599]

[52] Cheloufi S, Dos Santos CO, Chong MM, Hannon GJ. A dicer-independent miRNA biogenesis pathway that requires Ago catalysis. Nature 2010; 465(7298): 584-9.
[http://dx.doi.org/10.1038/nature09092] [PMID: 20424607]

[53] Cifuentes D, *et al.* A novel miRNA processing pathway independent of Dicer requires Argonaute2 catalytic activity. Scienc 2010; 328: 1694-8.
[http://dx.doi.org/10.1126/science.1190809]

[54] Yates LA, Norbury CJ, Gilbert RJ. The long and short of microRNA. Cell 2013; 153(3): 516-9.
[http://dx.doi.org/10.1016/j.cell.2013.04.003] [PMID: 23622238]

[55] Krol J, Loedige I, Filipowicz W. The widespread regulation of microRNA biogenesis, function and decay. Nature reviews 2010; 11: 597-610.
[http://dx.doi.org/10.1038/nrg2843]

[56] Meister G, Tuschl T. Mechanisms of gene silencing by double-stranded RNA. Nature 2004; 431(7006): 343-9.
[http://dx.doi.org/10.1038/nature02873] [PMID: 15372041]

[57] Brennecke J, Stark A, Russell RB, Cohen SM. Principles of microRNA-target recognition. PLoS Biol 2005; 3(3): e85.
[http://dx.doi.org/10.1371/journal.pbio.0030085] [PMID: 15723116]

[58] Grimson A, Farh KK, Johnston WK, Garrett-Engele P, Lim LP, Bartel DP. MicroRNA targeting specificity in mammals: determinants beyond seed pairing. Mol Cell 2007; 27(1): 91-105.
[http://dx.doi.org/10.1016/j.molcel.2007.06.017] [PMID: 17612493]

[59] Liu J. Control of protein synthesis and mRNA degradation by microRNAs. Curr Opin Cell Biol 2008; 20(2): 214-21.
[http://dx.doi.org/10.1016/j.ceb.2008.01.006] [PMID: 18329869]

[60] Guo H, Ingolia NT, Weissman JS, Bartel DP. Mammalian microRNAs predominantly act to decrease target mRNA levels. Nature 2010; 466(7308): 835-40.
[http://dx.doi.org/10.1038/nature09267] [PMID: 20703300]

[61] Salmena L, Poliseno L, Tay Y, Kats L, Pandolfi PP. A ceRNA hypothesis: the Rosetta Stone of a hidden RNA language? Cell 2011; 146(3): 353-8.
[http://dx.doi.org/10.1016/j.cell.2011.07.014] [PMID: 21802130]

[62] Tay Y, Kats L, Salmena L, *et al.* Coding-independent regulation of the tumor suppressor PTEN by competing endogenous mRNAs. Cell 2011; 147(2): 344-57.
[http://dx.doi.org/10.1016/j.cell.2011.09.029] [PMID: 22000013]

[63] Crown ED. The role of mitogen activated protein kinase signaling in microglia and neurons in the initiation and maintenance of chronic pain. Exp Neurol 2012; 234(2): 330-9.
[http://dx.doi.org/10.1016/j.expneurol.2011.10.019] [PMID: 22062045]

[64] Ji RR, Kohno T, Moore KA, Woolf CJ. Central sensitization and LTP: do pain and memory share similar mechanisms? Trends Neurosci 2003; 26(12): 696-705. [http://dx.doi.org/10.1016/j.tins.2003.09.017] [PMID: 14624855]

[65] Kusuda R, Cadetti F, Ravanelli MI, *et al.* Differential expression of microRNAs in mouse pain models. Mol Pain 2011; 7: 17. [http://dx.doi.org/10.1186/1744-8069-7-17] [PMID: 21385380]

[66] Tam Tam S, Bastian I, Zhou XF, *et al.* MicroRNA-143 expression in dorsal root ganglion neurons. Cell Tissue Res 2011; 346(2): 163-73. [http://dx.doi.org/10.1007/s00441-011-1263-x] [PMID: 22048787]

[67] Sakai A, Suzuki H. Nerve injury-induced upregulation of miR-21 in the primary sensory neurons contributes to neuropathic pain in rats. Biochem Biophys Res Commun 2013; 435(2): 176-81. [http://dx.doi.org/10.1016/j.bbrc.2013.04.089] [PMID: 23665014]

[68] Sakai A, Saitow F, Miyake N, Miyake K, Shimada T, Suzuki H. miR-7a alleviates the maintenance of neuropathic pain through regulation of neuronal excitability. Brain 2013; 136(Pt 9): 2738-50. [http://dx.doi.org/10.1093/brain/awt191] [PMID: 23861446]

[69] Bali KK, Selvaraj D, Satagopam VP, Lu J, Schneider R, Kuner R. Genome-wide identification and functional analyses of microRNA signatures associated with cancer pain. EMBO Mol Med 2013; 5(11): 1740-58. [http://dx.doi.org/10.1002/emmm.201302797] [PMID: 24039159]

[70] Zhao J, Lee MC, Momin A, *et al.* Small RNAs control sodium channel expression, nociceptor excitability, and pain thresholds. J Neurosci 2010; 30(32): 10860-71. [http://dx.doi.org/10.1523/JNEUROSCI.1980-10.2010] [PMID: 20702715]

[71] Xu Y, Zhang X, Pu S, Wu J, Lv Y, Du D. Circulating microRNA expression profile: a novel potential predictor for chronic nervous lesions. Acta Biochim Biophys Sin (Shanghai) 2014; 46(11): 942-9. [http://dx.doi.org/10.1093/abbs/gmu090] [PMID: 25274330]

[72] Bali KK, Hackenberg M, Lubin A, Kuner R, Devor M. Sources of individual variability: miRNAs that predispose to neuropathic pain identified using genome-wide sequencing. Mol Pain 2014; 10: 22. [http://dx.doi.org/10.1186/1744-8069-10-22] [PMID: 24642266]

[73] Gong Q, Lu Z, Huang Q, *et al.* Altered microRNAs expression profiling in mice with diabetic neuropathic pain. Biochem Biophys Res Commun 2015; 456(2): 615-20. [http://dx.doi.org/10.1016/j.bbrc.2014.12.004] [PMID: 25498543]

[74] Strickland IT, Richards L, Holmes FE, Wynick D, Uney JB, Wong LF. Axotomy-induced miR-21 promotes axon growth in adult dorsal root ganglion neurons. PLoS One 2011; 6(8): e23423. [http://dx.doi.org/10.1371/journal.pone.0023423] [PMID: 21853131]

[75] Zhou S, Shen D, Wang Y, *et al.* microRNA-222 targeting PTEN promotes neurite outgrowth from adult dorsal root ganglion neurons following sciatic nerve transection. PLoS One 2012; 7(9): e44768. [http://dx.doi.org/10.1371/journal.pone.0044768] [PMID: 23028614]

[76] Wu D, Murashov AK. MicroRNA-431 regulates axon regeneration in mature sensory neurons by targeting the Wnt antagonist Kremen1. Front Mol Neurosci 2013; 6: 35. [http://dx.doi.org/10.3389/fnmol.2013.00035] [PMID: 24167472]

[77] Lopez-Santiago LF, Pertin M, Morisod X, *et al.* Sodium channel beta2 subunits regulate tetrodotoxin-sensitive sodium channels in small dorsal root ganglion neurons and modulate the response to pain. J Neurosci 2006; 26(30): 7984-94.
[http://dx.doi.org/10.1523/JNEUROSCI.2211-06.2006] [PMID: 16870743]

[78] Xu S, Witmer PD, Lumayag S, Kovacs B, Valle D. MicroRNA (miRNA) transcriptome of mouse retina and identification of a sensory organ-specific miRNA cluster. J Biol Chem 2007; 282(34): 25053-66.
[http://dx.doi.org/10.1074/jbc.M700501200] [PMID: 17597072]

[79] Aldrich BT, Frakes EP, Kasuya J, Hammond DL, Kitamoto T. Changes in expression of sensory organ-specific microRNAs in rat dorsal root ganglia in association with mechanical hypersensitivity induced by spinal nerve ligation. Neuroscience 2009; 164(2): 711-23.
[http://dx.doi.org/10.1016/j.neuroscience.2009.08.033] [PMID: 19699278]

[80] Li X, Kroin JS, Kc R, *et al.* Altered spinal microRNA-146a and the microRNA-183 cluster contribute to osteoarthritic pain in knee joints. J Bone Miner Res 2013; 28(12): 2512-22.
[http://dx.doi.org/10.1002/jbmr.2002] [PMID: 23744481]

[81] Bai G, Ambalavanar R, Wei D, Dessem D. Downregulation of selective microRNAs in trigeminal ganglion neurons following inflammatory muscle pain. Mol Pain 2007; 3: 15.
[http://dx.doi.org/10.1186/1744-8069-3-15] [PMID: 17559665]

[82] Wu D, Raafat M, Pak E, Hammond S, Murashov AK. MicroRNA machinery responds to peripheral nerve lesion in an injury-regulated pattern. Neuroscience 2011; 190: 386-97.
[http://dx.doi.org/10.1016/j.neuroscience.2011.06.017] [PMID: 21689732]

[83] Yu B, Zhou S, Qian T, Wang Y, Ding F, Gu X. Altered microRNA expression following sciatic nerve resection in dorsal root ganglia of rats. Acta Biochim Biophys Sin (Shanghai) 2011; 43(11): 909-15.
[http://dx.doi.org/10.1093/abbs/gmr083] [PMID: 21908854]

[84] von Schack D, Agostino MJ, Murray BS, *et al.* Dynamic changes in the microRNA expression profile reveal multiple regulatory mechanisms in the spinal nerve ligation model of neuropathic pain. PLoS One 2011; 6(3): e17670.
[http://dx.doi.org/10.1371/journal.pone.0017670] [PMID: 21423802]

[85] Genda Y, Arai M, Ishikawa M, Tanaka S, Okabe T, Sakamoto A. microRNA changes in the dorsal horn of the spinal cord of rats with chronic constriction injury: A TaqMan® Low Density Array study. Int J Mol Med 2013; 31(1): 129-37.
[PMID: 23124577]

[86] Brandenburger T, Castoldi M, Brendel M, *et al.* Expression of spinal cord microRNAs in a rat model of chronic neuropathic pain. Neurosci Lett 2012; 506(2): 281-6.
[http://dx.doi.org/10.1016/j.neulet.2011.11.023] [PMID: 22138088]

[87] Li H, Huang Y, Ma C, Yu X, Zhang Z, Shen L. MiR-203 involves in neuropathic pain development and represses Rap1a expression in nerve growth factor differentiated neuronal PC12 cells. Clin J Pain 2015; 31(1): 36-43.
[http://dx.doi.org/10.1097/AJP.0000000000000070] [PMID: 24451631]

[88] Nakanishi K, Nakasa T, Tanaka N, *et al.* Responses of microRNAs 124a and 223 following spinal

cord injury in mice. Spinal Cord 2010; 48(3): 192-6.
[http://dx.doi.org/10.1038/sc.2009.89] [PMID: 19621023]

[89] Li X, Gibson G, Kim JS, *et al.* MicroRNA-146a is linked to pain-related pathophysiology of osteoarthritis. Gene 2011; 480(1-2): 34-41.
[http://dx.doi.org/10.1016/j.gene.2011.03.003] [PMID: 21397669]

[90] Willemen HL, Huo XJ, Mao-Ying QL, Zijlstra J, Heijnen CJ, Kavelaars A. MicroRNA-124 as a novel treatment for persistent hyperalgesia. J Neuroinflammation 2012; 9: 143.
[http://dx.doi.org/10.1186/1742-2094-9-143] [PMID: 22731384]

[91] Favereaux A, Thoumine O, Bouali-Benazzouz R, *et al.* Bidirectional integrative regulation of Cav1.2 calcium channel by microRNA miR-103: role in pain. EMBO J 2011; 30(18): 3830-41.
[http://dx.doi.org/10.1038/emboj.2011.249] [PMID: 21804529]

[92] Kynast KL, Russe OQ, Möser CV, Geisslinger G, Niederberger E. Modulation of central nervous system-specific microRNA-124a alters the inflammatory response in the formalin test in mice. Pain 2013; 154(3): 368-76.
[http://dx.doi.org/10.1016/j.pain.2012.11.010] [PMID: 23318130]

[93] Arai M, *et al.* The miRNA and mRNA changes in rat hippocampi after chronic constriction injury. Pain medicine 2013; 14: 720-9.
[http://dx.doi.org/10.1111/pme.12066]

[94] Hori Y, Goto G, Arai-Iwasaki M, Ishikawa M, Sakamoto A. Differential expression of rat hippocampal microRNAs in two rat models of chronic pain. Int J Mol Med 2013; 32(6): 1287-92.
[PMID: 24065306]

[95] Imai S, Saeki M, Yanase M, *et al.* Change in microRNAs associated with neuronal adaptive responses in the nucleus accumbens under neuropathic pain. J Neurosci 2011; 31(43): 15294-9.
[http://dx.doi.org/10.1523/JNEUROSCI.0921-11.2011] [PMID: 22031875]

[96] Bär KJ, Wagner G, Koschke M, *et al.* Increased prefrontal activation during pain perception in major depression. Biol Psychiatry 2007; 62(11): 1281-7.
[http://dx.doi.org/10.1016/j.biopsych.2007.02.011] [PMID: 17570347]

[97] Poh KW, Yeo JF, Ong WY. MicroRNA changes in the mouse prefrontal cortex after inflammatory pain. European journal of pain 2011; 15(801): e1-e12.

[98] He Y, Yang C, Kirkmire CM, Wang ZJ. Regulation of opioid tolerance by let-7 family microRNA targeting the mu opioid receptor. J Neurosci 2010; 30(30): 10251-8.
[http://dx.doi.org/10.1523/JNEUROSCI.2419-10.2010] [PMID: 20668208]

[99] Park CK, Xu ZZ, Berta T, *et al.* Extracellular microRNAs activate nociceptor neurons to elicit pain *via* TLR7 and TRPA1. Neuron 2014; 82(1): 47-54.
[http://dx.doi.org/10.1016/j.neuron.2014.02.011] [PMID: 24698267]

[100] Orlova IA, Alexander GM, Qureshi RA, *et al.* MicroRNA modulation in complex regional pain syndrome. J Transl Med 2011; 9: 195.
[http://dx.doi.org/10.1186/1479-5876-9-195] [PMID: 22074333]

[101] Valencia-Sanchez MA, Liu J, Hannon GJ, Parker R. Control of translation and mRNA degradation by miRNAs and siRNAs. Genes Dev 2006; 20(5): 515-24.

[http://dx.doi.org/10.1101/gad.1399806] [PMID: 16510870]

[102] John B, Enright AJ, Aravin A, Tuschl T, Sander C, Marks DS. Human MicroRNA targets. PLoS Biol 2004; 2(11): e363.
[http://dx.doi.org/10.1371/journal.pbio.0020363] [PMID: 15502875]

[103] Rehmsmeier M, *et al.* Fast and effective prediction of microRNA/target duplexes. RNA 2004; 10: 1507-7.

[104] Lewis BP, Burge CB, Bartel DP. Conserved seed pairing, often flanked by adenosines, indicates that thousands of human genes are microRNA targets. Cell 2005; 120(1): 15-20.
[http://dx.doi.org/10.1016/j.cell.2004.12.035] [PMID: 15652477]

[105] Kuhn DE, *et al.* Experimental validation of miRNA targets. Methods (San Diego, Calif) 2008; 44: 47-54.
[http://dx.doi.org/10.1016/j.ymeth.2007.09.005]

[106] Davis S, Lollo B, Freier S, Esau C. Improved targeting of miRNA with antisense oligonucleotides. Nucleic Acids Res 2006; 34(8): 2294-304.
[http://dx.doi.org/10.1093/nar/gkl183] [PMID: 16690972]

[107] Obad S, dos Santos CO, Petri A, *et al.* Silencing of microRNA families by seed-targeting tiny LNAs. Nat Genet 2011; 43(4): 371-8.
[http://dx.doi.org/10.1038/ng.786] [PMID: 21423181]

[108] Stenvang J, Petri A, Lindow M, Obad S, Kauppinen S. Inhibition of microRNA function by antimiR oligonucleotides. Silence 2012; 3(1): 1.
[http://dx.doi.org/10.1186/1758-907X-3-1] [PMID: 22230293]

[109] Elmén J, Lindow M, Schütz S, *et al.* LNA-mediated microRNA silencing in non-human primates. Nature 2008; 452(7189): 896-9.
[http://dx.doi.org/10.1038/nature06783] [PMID: 18368051]

[110] Krützfeldt J, Rajewsky N, Braich R, *et al.* Silencing of microRNAs *in vivo* with 'antagomirs'. Nature 2005; 438(7068): 685-9.
[http://dx.doi.org/10.1038/nature04303] [PMID: 16258535]

[111] Cheng HY, Papp JW, Varlamova O, *et al.* microRNA modulation of circadian-clock period and entrainment. Neuron 2007; 54(5): 813-29.
[http://dx.doi.org/10.1016/j.neuron.2007.05.017] [PMID: 17553428]

[112] Janssen HL, Reesink HW, Lawitz EJ, *et al.* Treatment of HCV infection by targeting microRNA. N Engl J Med 2013; 368(18): 1685-94.
[http://dx.doi.org/10.1056/NEJMoa1209026] [PMID: 23534542]

[113] Rayner KJ, Esau CC, Hussain FN, *et al.* Inhibition of miR-33a/b in non-human primates raises plasma HDL and lowers VLDL triglycerides. Nature 2011; 478(7369): 404-7.
[http://dx.doi.org/10.1038/nature10486] [PMID: 22012398]

[114] Tappe A, Klugmann M, Luo C, *et al.* Synaptic scaffolding protein Homer1a protects against chronic inflammatory pain. Nat Med 2006; 12(6): 677-81.
[http://dx.doi.org/10.1038/nm1406] [PMID: 16715092]

[115] Terashima T, Oka K, Kritz AB, Kojima H, Baker AH, Chan L. DRG-targeted helper-dependent adenoviruses mediate selective gene delivery for therapeutic rescue of sensory neuronopathies in mice. J Clin Invest 2009; 119(7): 2100-12.
[PMID: 19603551]

[116] Ebert MS, Neilson JR, Sharp PA. MicroRNA sponges: competitive inhibitors of small RNAs in mammalian cells. Nat Methods 2007; 4(9): 721-6.
[http://dx.doi.org/10.1038/nmeth1079] [PMID: 17694064]

[117] Park CY, Choi YS, McManus MT. Analysis of microRNA knockouts in mice. Hum Mol Genet 2010; 19(R2): R169-75.
[http://dx.doi.org/10.1093/hmg/ddq367] [PMID: 20805106]

[118] Prosser HM, Koike-Yusa H, Cooper JD, Law FC, Bradley A. A resource of vectors and ES cells for targeted deletion of microRNAs in mice. Nat Biotechnol 2011; 29(9): 840-5.
[http://dx.doi.org/10.1038/nbt.1929] [PMID: 21822254]

[119] Ghosh R, Singh LC, Shohet JM, Gunaratne PH. A gold nanoparticle platform for the delivery of functional microRNAs into cancer cells. Biomaterials 2013; 34(3): 807-16.
[http://dx.doi.org/10.1016/j.biomaterials.2012.10.023] [PMID: 23111335]

[120] Crew E, Tessel MA, Rahman S, *et al.* MicroRNA conjugated gold nanoparticles and cell transfection. Anal Chem 2012; 84(1): 26-9.
[http://dx.doi.org/10.1021/ac202749p] [PMID: 22148593]

[121] Li J, Chen YC, Tseng YC, Mozumdar S, Huang L. Biodegradable calcium phosphate nanoparticle with lipid coating for systemic siRNA delivery. J Control Release 2010; 142(3): 416-21.
[http://dx.doi.org/10.1016/j.jconrel.2009.11.008] [PMID: 19919845]

[122] Pramanik D, Campbell NR, Karikari C, *et al.* Restitution of tumor suppressor microRNAs using a systemic nanovector inhibits pancreatic cancer growth in mice. Mol Cancer Ther 2011; 10(8): 1470-80.
[http://dx.doi.org/10.1158/1535-7163.MCT-11-0152] [PMID: 21622730]

[123] Alvarez-Erviti L, Seow Y, Yin H, Betts C, Lakhal S, Wood MJ. Delivery of siRNA to the mouse brain by systemic injection of targeted exosomes. Nat Biotechnol 2011; 29(4): 341-5.
[http://dx.doi.org/10.1038/nbt.1807] [PMID: 21423189]

[124] Lin CR, Chen KH, Yang CH, Huang HW, Sheen-Chen SM. Intrathecal miR-183 delivery suppresses mechanical allodynia in mononeuropathic rats. Eur J Neurosci 2014; 39(10): 1682-9.
[http://dx.doi.org/10.1111/ejn.12522] [PMID: 24612023]

[125] Chen HP, Zhou W, Kang LM, *et al.* Intrathecal miR-96 inhibits Nav1.3 expression and alleviates neuropathic pain in rat following chronic construction injury. Neurochem Res 2014; 39(1): 76-83.
[http://dx.doi.org/10.1007/s11064-013-1192-z] [PMID: 24234845]

[126] Ni J, Gao Y, Gong S, Guo S, Hisamitsu T, Jiang X. Regulation of μ-opioid type 1 receptors by microRNA134 in dorsal root ganglion neurons following peripheral inflammation. Eur J Pain 2013; 17(3): 313-23.
[http://dx.doi.org/10.1002/j.1532-2149.2012.00197.x] [PMID: 22865422]

[127] Liu NK, Wang XF, Lu QB, Xu XM. Altered microRNA expression following traumatic spinal cord

injury. Exp Neurol 2009; 219(2): 424-9.
[http://dx.doi.org/10.1016/j.expneurol.2009.06.015] [PMID: 19576215]

[128] Bhalala OG, Pan L, Sahni V, *et al.* microRNA-21 regulates astrocytic response following spinal cord injury. J Neurosci 2012; 32(50): 17935-47.
[http://dx.doi.org/10.1523/JNEUROSCI.3860-12.2012] [PMID: 23238710]

[129] Im YB, Jee MK, Choi JI, Cho HT, Kwon OH, Kang SK. Molecular targeting of NOX4 for neuropathic pain after traumatic injury of the spinal cord. Cell Death Dis 2012; 3: e426.
[http://dx.doi.org/10.1038/cddis.2012.168] [PMID: 23152062]

[130] Shi G, Shi J, Liu K, *et al.* Increased miR-195 aggravates neuropathic pain by inhibiting autophagy following peripheral nerve injury. Glia 2013; 61(4): 504-12.
[http://dx.doi.org/10.1002/glia.22451] [PMID: 23361941]

[131] Wu D, Raafat A, Pak E, Clemens S, Murashov AK. Dicer-microRNA pathway is critical for peripheral nerve regeneration and functional recovery *in vivo* and regenerative axonogenesis *in vitro.* Exp Neurol 2012; 233(1): 555-65.
[http://dx.doi.org/10.1016/j.expneurol.2011.11.041] [PMID: 22178326]

[132] Yu B, Zhou S, Hu W, *et al.* Altered long noncoding RNA expressions in dorsal root ganglion after rat sciatic nerve injury. Neurosci Lett 2013; 534: 117-22.
[http://dx.doi.org/10.1016/j.neulet.2012.12.014] [PMID: 23274483]

[133] Huang Y, Yang YB, Zhang XH, Yu XL, Wang ZB, Cheng XC. MicroRNA-21 gene and cancer. Med Oncol 2013; 30(1): 376.
[http://dx.doi.org/10.1007/s12032-012-0376-8] [PMID: 23277281]

[134] Kawasaki Y, Xu ZZ, Wang X, *et al.* Distinct roles of matrix metalloproteases in the early- and late-phase development of neuropathic pain. Nat Med 2008; 14(3): 331-6.
[http://dx.doi.org/10.1038/nm1723] [PMID: 18264108]

[135] Meng F, Henson R, Wehbe-Janek H, Ghoshal K, Jacob ST, Patel T. MicroRNA-21 regulates expression of the PTEN tumor suppressor gene in human hepatocellular cancer. Gastroenterology 2007; 133(2): 647-58.
[http://dx.doi.org/10.1053/j.gastro.2007.05.022] [PMID: 17681183]

[136] Wiech K, Kalisch R, Weiskopf N, Pleger B, Stephan KE, Dolan RJ. Anterolateral prefrontal cortex mediates the analgesic effect of expected and perceived control over pain. J Neurosci 2006; 26(44): 11501-9.
[http://dx.doi.org/10.1523/JNEUROSCI.2568-06.2006] [PMID: 17079679]

CHAPTER 7

The Ameliorative Potential of 7-Hydroxy-4-Methylcoumarin in Acrylamide Induced Neuropathic Pain *via* Improving of Mitochondrial Function in Rat

Jaspreet Kaur, Arunachalam Muthuraman* and **Muthusamy Ramesh**

Neuropharmacology Division, Department of Pharmacology and Toxicology, Akal College of Pharmacy & technical Education, Mastuana Sahib, Sangrur 148002, Punjab, India

Abstract: The present study was designed to investigate the analgesic potential of 7-hydroxy-4-methylcoumarin (HMC) in acrylamide induced neuropathic pain in rats. Acrylamide (30 mg/kg, *i.p.*; once in three days, for 24 consecutive days) was administered for inducing neuropathic pain. The acrylamide induced nociceptive pain sensation, *i.e.,* acetone drop, plantar, hot plate, Von Frey Hair and tail immersion tests have been assessed at different time intervals, *i.e.,* 0, 6, 12, 18 and 24th day. Furthermore, the biochemical estimation, *i.e.,* thiobarbituric acid reactive substances (TBARS), reduced glutathione (GSH), total calcium, cytochrome c oxidase activity and ATP content levels were estimated from the sciatic nerve tissue sample on 24th day. The HMC (10 and 20 mg/kg, *p.o.*) and cyclosporin A (CsA, 50 µM/kg; *p.o.*) was administered for 24 consecutive days, one hour before each injection of acrylamide. The treatment of acrylamide resulted in significant ($P < 0.05$) changes of behavioral and biochemical changes. Pretreatment of HMC ameliorate the acrylamide induced changes of behavioral and biochemical parameters in a dose dependent manner. These results are similar to that of CsA treated group. Based on these findings, it may conclude that, HMC possesses the potential ameliorative effect against acrylamide induced neuropathic pain, it may be because of its therapeutic potential of anti-oxidant, anti-lipidperoxidative, calcium ion regulatory and mitochondrial permeability transition pore inhibitory action.

* **Coresponding author Arunachalam Muthuraman:** Neuropharmacology Division, Department of Pharmacology and Toxicology, Akal College of Pharmacy & technical Education, Mastuana Sahib, Sangrur 148002, Punjab, India. E-mail: arunachalammu@gmail.com

Puneetpal Singh (Ed.)

Keywords: 7-hydroxy-4-methylcoumarin, Acrylamide, Adenosine triphosphate, Allodynia, Calcium, Cyclosporin A, Cytochrome c oxidase, Electron transport chain, Hyperalgesia, Mitochondrial dysfunction.

INTRODUCTION

According to the International Association for the Study of Pain (IASP), neuropathic pain is defined as *"pain initiated or caused by a primary lesion or dysfunction or transitory perturbation in the peripheral or central nervous system"* [1]. It is characterized by affecting the somatosensory system leading to produce the spontaneous pain, hyperalgesia, hypothesia, dysthesia and allodynia [2]. In addition, the Food and Drug Administration (FDA) approved few drugs to manage the neuropathic pain syndrome, *i.e.,* anti-convulsants, anti-depressants, topical medicines and opioids [3, 4]. However, these medications give partially relief from the symptoms, induce wide spectrum of adverse effects and lack specificity. Thus, clinical usage of these drugs is limited in the management of neuropathic pain [5, 6]. The various animal models are well established for evaluating newer agents in the management of neuropathic pain syndrome. Acrylamide is one of the chemical methods for inducing neuropathic pain [7].

Acrylamide (prop-2-enamide) is an odourless white crystalline solid. It is widely used in various chemical industries for preparing polyacrylamides, water-soluble thickeners, sugar manufacturing, pesticide formulations, preparing permanent cement, press fabrics/plastic products, dyes and ore processing [8, 9]. It is also used as binding, thickening / flocculating agent, cosmetic preparation and gel electrophoresis process in pharmaceutical science [10, 11]. In addition, acrylamide was found in many roasted starchy foods [12 - 14]. Furthermore, it is present in black olives, prunes, dried pears, coffee, cocoa powder, roasted almonds, whole wheat bread and Pringles [14, 15]. The precise mechanism of acrylamide formation in foods remains unclear, but it is believed that, it is a byproduct of the Maillard reaction between asparagine and reducing sugars (*i.e.,* fructose and glucose) or reactive carbonyls at temperatures above 120 °C [16, 17]. Various studies have reported that, acrylamide is known to have potential neurotoxic effect [18, 19]. In fact, it produces the potential distal multifocal axonal degeneration, which is also known as "dying back" neuropathy. Generally, dying back" neuropathy is a progressive loss of peripheral and central neuronal axon which is observed in both humans as well as animal species [20 - 22]. Acrylamide (30 mg/kg, *i.p.,* for 24 consecutive days) induced neuropathic pain is one of the common experimental models of the neuropathic pain disorder. It is a clinically relevant model for neurotoxic chemical associated neuropathic pain and is widely accepted model due to its similar pathophysiological mechanism in humans as well as in rodents [20, 23].

Recently, various herbal constituents are employed in the management of neuropathic pain, *i.e.,* quercetin [24]; geraniol and curcumin [25]; safranal [26]; puerarin [27]; thymoquinone [28] which have been documented to produce the attenuation of neuropathic pain. Coumarin is one of the important flavonoid in herbal plants [24]. Higher concentrations of coumarin are present in *Dipteryx odorata*, *Anthoxanthum odoratum*, *Galium odoratum* and *Albizia antunesiana* [29, 30]. It has various pharmacological actions such as anti-diabetic [31], hepatoprotection [32], anti-coagulant [33], anti-tumor, and anti-fungal activity [34, 35]. Coumarin is one of the major constituents of the various herbal plants and has various therapeutic actions against ulcerative colitis [36], psychosis [37], thrombosis [38] and diabetes [39]. Recently, various reports have documented that, coumarin derivatives also possess the potential pharmacological actions, *i.e.,* anti-cancer [40], anti-inflammation [41] and improvement of learning and memory function [42]. The molecular mechanism of coumarin is known to have the free radical scavenger, *i.e.,* reactive oxygen species, reactive nitrogen species and reactive chlorine species, calcium channel blocking actions [43].

Furthermore, coumarin derivative is known to possess the potential action on mitochondrial functional regulation [44]. In addition, cyclosporine A is also documented to produce the neuroprotection *via* regulation of mitochondrial function by inhibition of mitochondrial permeability transition pore (MPTP) opening and release of cytochrome c [45]. Thus, cyclosporine A served as positive control in this study. Acrylamide is known to cause the mitochondrial dysfunction in the nervous system *via* opening of MPTP [46, 47]. Therefore, the present study has been designed to investigate the molecular mechanism and therapeutic potential of 7-hydroxy-4-methylcoumarin in acrylamide induced neuropathic pain in rats.

MATERIALS AND METHODS

Drugs and Chemicals

Acrylamide was purchased from CDH, New Delhi. The gift sample of Cyclosporin A was obtained as a gift from Novartis Pvt. Ltd., Mumbai, India. 1,1',3,3' tetramethoxy propane and Folin-Ciocalteus phenol reagent (Merck Limited, Mumbai), [5,5'-dithio, bis-(2-nitrobenzoic acid)] (DTNB), reduced glutathione, bovine serum albumin, (Sisco Research Laboratories Pvt. Ltd. Mumbai) and thio-barbituric acid (Loba Chem. Mumbai), were procured for the present study. DTNB was dissolved in 1% w/v of sodium citrate. All other reagents were used as an analytical grade and obtained from SD Fine chemicals, Mumbai, India.

Animals

Wistar rats (either sex, 150-200 gm) were employed in the present study. Animals were maintained with standard laboratory diet (Markfed cotton seed processing plant, Gidderbaha, Mukatsar, Punjab, India) and allowed to free access of water *ad libitum*. They were housed in the animal house and exposed to 12 hour light and dark. The experimental protocol was duly approved by the Institutional Animal Ethical Committee and animals were maintained as per guidelines of the Committee for the Purpose of Control and Supervision of Experiments on Animals (ATRC/14/13), Ministery of Environment and Forest, Government of India (Reg. no.: 1407/a/11/CPCSEA).

Induction of Neuropathic Pain

The neuropathic pain was induced by intraperitoneal (*i.p.*) injection of acrylamide following method described by Gold *et al.* [48] with slight modification of Ling *et al.* [23]. Briefly the acrylamide (30 mg/kg; *i.p.,* once in three days) was administered briefly for 24 consecutive days. All the groups of animals were subjected to assess nociceptive threshold at different time intervals, *i.e.,* 0, 6, 12, 18 and 24th day.

Assessment of Behavioral Pain Sensation

The animals were subjected to the assessment of behavioral tests such as acetone drop, plantar, hot plate, Von Frey hair and tail immersion tests as thermal allodynia, thermal hyperalgesia and mechanical allodynia in paw and thermal hyperalgesia was observed in tail respectively. The order of tests was performed from low intensity to a higher intensity of stimuli. These tests explored the nociceptive pain sensation in peripheral (paw region) as well as in central (tail region) nervous system.

Acetone Drop Test

The cold chemical sensitivity (allodynia) of the right hind paw was assessed as described by the method of Choi *et al.* [49]. Briefly, the rats were placed on the top of a wire mesh grid, allowing access to the hind paws. The acclimatization period of 5 minutes was maintained. Acetone (100 μl) was sprayed on the plantar surface of the right hind paw of rat. The cold chemical sensitive reaction was observed for 1 minute and scored (*i.e.* score 1 for paw licking; score 2 for shaking; score 3 for right hind paw lifting duration below 4 second; score 4 for right hind paw lifting duration 5 to 8 second and scores 5 for right hind paw lifting duration 8 to 12 second), the total score was noted as 15; the highest score with respect to severe injury and the lowest score with respect to neuroprotection.

Plantar Test

The radiant heat sensitivity (hyperalgesia) of the right hind paw was assessed as described by the method of Hargreaves *et al.* [50]. Briefly, the hind paw of rat was placed on the radiant heat source of Hargreaves apparatus. The thermal sensitivity of the hind paw was observed as hind paw withdrawal latency from the radiant heat lamp source. Withdrawal of the hind limb was considered as positive response. The cut off time was maintained for 20 second.

Hot Plate Test

The conduction heat sensitivity (hyperalgesia) of the right hind paw was assessed as described by the method of Eddy *et al.* [51] with slight modification for assessing noxious thermal sensation. Briefly, the rat was placed on the top of a preheated (52 ± 0.5 °C) hot plate surface, allowing access to the paw licking or vocalization or jumping, whichever is first appearing to the nociceptive pain threshold. The cut- off time of 20 s was maintained to avoid the tissue injury.

Von Frey Hair Test

The mechanical touch sensitivity (allodynia) of the right hind paw was assessed as described by the method of Chaplan *et al.* [52]. Briefly, a calibrated nylon filament was selected based on the response of normal rat, which produced the minimum number withdrawal of the hind paw against 12 stimulus within 120 seconds (interval between each stimuli is 12 seconds). Minimum number of withdrawal of right hind paw of rats produced by the filament (No.: with a pending force of 4.6 g) was selected for further evaluation. The selected filament was applied to all the animals of the experimental group. A brisk withdrawal of the right hind limb was considered a positive response. The percentage response was calculated by the filament evoking a withdrawal threshold of the right hind paw 12 times out of 12 stimuli, *e.g.*, if the animal responds the six time hind paw withdrawal equal to 50% response.

Tail Immersion Test

The spinal nociceptive pain sensitivity (hyperalgesia) was assessed in the tail region as described method of Necker and Hellon [53]. Briefly, tip of the rat's tail, *i.e.,* 1 cm level from the terminal part of the tail was immersed into the temperature (52 ± 0.05 °C) controlled water chamber. Spinal thermal hyperalgesia was assessed by the time taken for withdrawal of the tail (*i.e.,* flick response) from water bath as indicated tail withdrawal reflex. The cut off time of 15 seconds was maintained to avoid the tissue injury.

Estimation of Tissue Biomarkers Changes

All the groups of animals were sacrificed after completion of the 24th day behavioral assessment by cervical dislocation method and the sciatic nerve was isolated immediately. The sciatic nerve homogenate (10% w/v) was prepared with 0.1 M Tris-HCL buffer (PH-7.4) and centrifuged with 2000 g, for 10 min, at 4 °C [54]. The supernatant was used for the estimation of tissue total protein, thiobarbituric acid reactive substances (TBARS) and reduced glutathione (GSH) content. For the estimation of tissue total calcium, the homogenate was prepared with triple distilled water. The pellet was used for the isolation of mitochondria of the sciatic nerve and used for the estimation of cytochrome c oxidase activity and ATP content.

Estimation of Total Protein Content

The tissue total protein content was estimated as described by the method of Lowry *et al.* [55]. Briefly, 300 µl of supernatant was diluted up to 1 ml with distilled water in a test tube. The 5 ml of Lowry's reagent was added and allowed to stand for 15 min at room temperature. Then 0.5 ml of Folin-Ciocalteu reagent was added and the contents were vortexed vigorously and incubated at room temperature for 30 min. This reaction gives a purple chromogen in the presence of protein. The protein content was determined spectrophotometrically (UV-1800 UV-Vis spectrophotometer, SHIMADZU Corporation, Tokyo, Japan) at 750 nm wavelength. The bovine serum albumin (1-10 mg) was used as standard. The results of total protein concentration were expressed as mg/ml of supernatant.

Estimation of Thiobarbituric Acid Reactive Substances (TBARS)

The tissue TBARS content was estimated as described by the method of Niehaus & Samuelsson [56]. Briefly, 0.5 ml tissue homogenate was mixed with 2.5 ml of (10%, w/v) trichloroacetic acid (TCA) solution and placed in a boiling water bath for 15 min. The test tubes were cooled at room temperature and centrifuged at 1500 rpm for 10 min. The 2 ml of each supernatant was transferred to a test tube containing 1 ml of trichloroacetic acid (TCA) (5% w/v) – thiobarbituric acid (TBA) (0.38% w/v) - HCl (0.25 N) mixture. Tubes were again placed in a boiling water bath for 15 min and cooled at room temperature. This reaction gives a pink chromogen in the presence of malondialdehyde. The absorbance changes in the tissue samples were measured by spectrophotometrically at 535 nm wavelength. The 1,1',3,3'-tetramethoxypropane (1-10 nmol) was used as standard. The results of TBARS were expressed as nmol of malondialdehyde/mg of protein.

Estimation of Reduced Glutathione (GSH) Content

The tissue GSH content was estimated as described by the method of Beutler *et al.* [57]. Briefly, 0.5 ml tissue homogenate was mixed with 2 ml of (0.3 M) disodium hydrogen phosphate solution and 0.25 ml of (0.001 M) freshly prepared 5,5'- dithiobis-2-nitrobenzoic acid (DTNB) solution. This reaction gives a yellow chromogen in the presence of GSH. The absorbance changes in the tissue samples were measured by spectrophotometrically at 412 nm wavelength. The GSH (10-100 μmol) was used as standard. The results of GSH were expressed as μmol of GSH/mg of protein.

Estimation of Total Calcium

Total calcium levels were estimated from the sciatic nerve tissue by the atomic emission spectroscopic method of Severinghaus & Ferrebee [58] with slight modification of Muthuraman *et al.* [54]. Briefly, the sciatic nerve tissue homogenate was mixed with 1 ml of trichloroacetic acid (4%) in ice cold conditions and centrifuged at 2000 rpm for 10 minutes. The clear supernatant was used for the estimation of total calcium ion by atomic emission spectroscopy at 556 nm. The mechanism of calcium ion estimation is due to the changes of color intensity in the flame, which shows free calcium ion concentration. The calcium chloride (0-1000 ppm) was used as standard. The results of total calcium were expressed as ppm of calcium/mg of protein.

Assessment of Mitochondrial Function

Preparation of Mitochondria

The mitochondria of sciatic nerve were isolated from the rat heart tissue as described by the method of Viader *et al.* [59] with slight modification of Frezza *et al.* [60]. Briefly, tissues were dissected and digested with collagenase for 20 min. Then, the sciatic nerve was homogenized for 2 minutes (Teflon-glass homogenizer, IMCORP, Ambala Cantt, India) at 2000 rpm for 10 min with homogenization buffer. The homogenization buffer contains 0.22 M mannitol, 70 mM sucrose, 10 mM Tris-HCl, 0.5 mM ethylenediamainetetraacetic acid (EDTA), 1mM ethylene-bis (oxythylenenitrilo) tetraacetic acid (EGTA) and 0.5% w/v bovine serum albumin (BSA) at pH 7.4. The clarified supernatant was centrifuged at 8000 g for 10 min. The pellet was resuspended in 1 ml of homogenization buffer without BSA and centrifuged at 7500g. The resulting pellet was resuspended once again in 250 μl of homogenization buffer without BSA. The protein concentration of the resuspended mitochondrial fractions was determined using Lowry's method. Five micrograms of protein from these mitochondrial preparations were used for further estimation of cytochrome c oxidase activity and adenosine triphosphate (ATP) content.

Estimation of Cytochrome C Oxidase Activity and ATP Content

The activity of cytochrome c oxidase was estimated according to the method of Rustin *et al.* [61]. The absorbance of the reaction mixture was measured spectrophotometrically at λ^{550} nm with λ^{580} nm as the reference wavelength (ε = 19.1 mM^{-1} cm^{-1} at 25°C for 10 min). The activity of cytochrome c oxidase was expressed in the terms of nanomole (nM) of cytochrome c oxidase activity per minute per mg of protein. ATP content was estimated by using HPLC technique as described by the method of Ally and Park [62], after neutralization of acid supernatant with sodium bicarbonate. The ATP level was expressed as picomole (pM) of ATP per mg of protein.

Experimental Protocol

Seven groups, each comprising six Wistar rats were employed in the present study.

Group I (Normal Control): Rats were not subjected to any drug, chemical and vehicle administration and kept for 24 consecutive days. The nociceptive pain threshold was assessed on different time intervals, *i.e.,* 0, 6, 12, 18 and 24th day. On the 24th day biochemical parameters *i.e.* total protein, TBARS, GSH, total calcium, cytochrome c oxidase activity and ATP content were estimated on the sciatic nerve tissue sample.

Group II (Acrylamide Treated Group): Rats were subjected to the administration of acrylamide (30 mg/kg; *i.p.,* once in three days) for 24 consecutive days. Behavioral and biochemical evaluations were carried out as described in group 1.

Group III (Vehicle Treated Group): Rats were subjected to the administration of normal saline (5 ml/kg of 0.5% w/v of carboxy methyl cellulose; *p.o.*) in acrylamide treated animals for 24 consecutive days. Behavioral and biochemical evaluations were carried out as described in group 1.

Group IV (HMC 20 mg/kg, per se Treated Group): Rats were subjected to the administration of 7-hydroxy-4-methylcoumarin (HMC 20 mg/kg; *p.o.*) in normal rats for 24 consecutive days. Behavioral and biochemical evaluations were carried out as described in group 1.

Group V-VI (HMC 10 and 20 mg/kg Treated Group): Rats were subjected to the administration of 7-hydroxy-4-methylcoumarin (HMC 20 mg/kg; *p.o.*) in acrylamide treated animals for 24 consecutive days. Behavioral and biochemical evaluations were carried out as described in group 1.

Group VII (Cyclosporin A 50 μM/kg, Treated Group): Rats were subjected to the administration of Cyclosporin A (CsA, 50 μM/kg; *p.o.*) in acrylamide treated animals for 24 consecutive days. Behavioral and biochemical evaluations were carried out as described in group 1.

Statistical Analysis

All the results were expressed as mean ± standard deviation (SD). Data obtained from behavioral tests were analyzed using two-way analysis of variance (ANOVA) followed by Bonferonni's post-hoc analysis. The data of tissue biomarkers *i.e.* total protein, TBARS, GSH, cytochrome c oxidase activity and ATP levels were analyzed using one way ANOVA followed by Tukey's multiple range tests for post-hoc analysis by using Sigmastat Version-3.5 software. A probability value of $P < 0.05$ was considered to be statistically significant.

RESULTS

Effect of HMC on Acetone Drop Test

The administration of acrylamide (30 mg/kg) resulted in a significant development of cold chemical allodynia as indicated by the rise in cold sensation score after the 6th day of acrylamide intoxication when compared to a normal control group. Administration of HMC (10 and 20 mg/kg) attenuated acrylamide induced rise in the cold chemical sensation in a dose dependent manner. Treatment of cyclosporin A (CsA, 50 µM/kg) also produced similar effects. However, HMC *per se* and vehicle treated group did not show any significant ($P < 0.05$) changes in acrylamide induced cold chemical sensation (Fig. **1**).

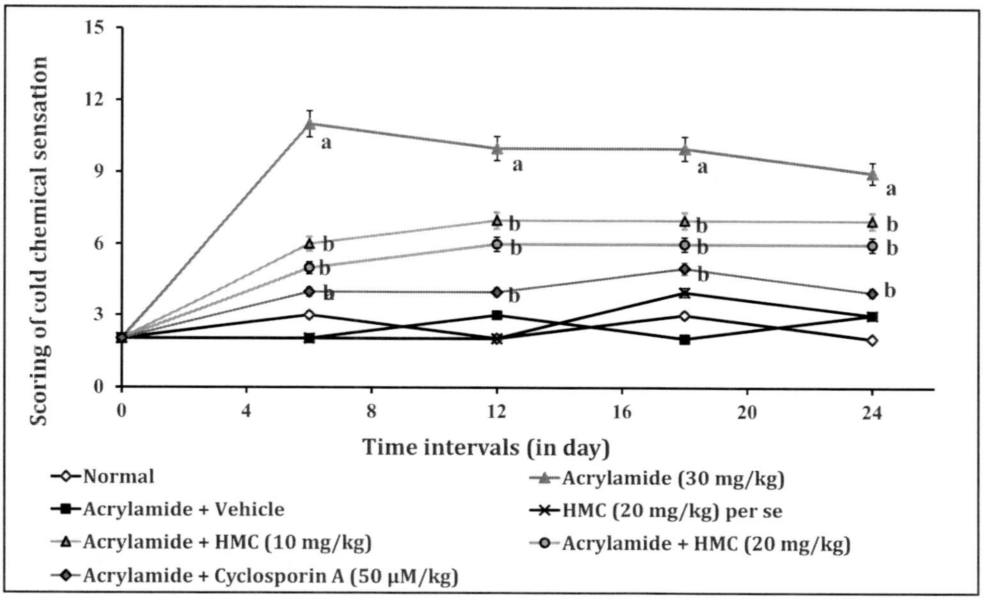

Fig. (1). Effect of HMC on acetone drop test.
HMC, 7-hydroxy-4-methylcoumarin.
Data were expressed as mean ± SD, six animal per group (n=6) were used for the statistical analysis.
[a]$P < 0.05$ *versus* normal control group.
[b]$P < 0.05$ *versus* acrylamide control group.

Effect of HMC on Plantar Test

The administration of acrylamide (30 mg/kg) resulted in a significant development of radiant heat hyperalgesia as indicated by a decrease in right hind paw withdrawal threshold after the 6th day of acrylamide intoxication when compared to a normal control group. Administration of HMC (10 and 20 mg/kg) attenuated acrylamide induced decrease in the thermal nociceptive pain threshold in a dose dependent manner. Treatment of cyclosporin A (CsA, 50 μM/kg) also produced similar effects. However, HMC *per se* and vehicle treated group did not show any significant ($P > 0.05$) changes in acrylamide induced thermal hyperalgesia (Fig. **2**).

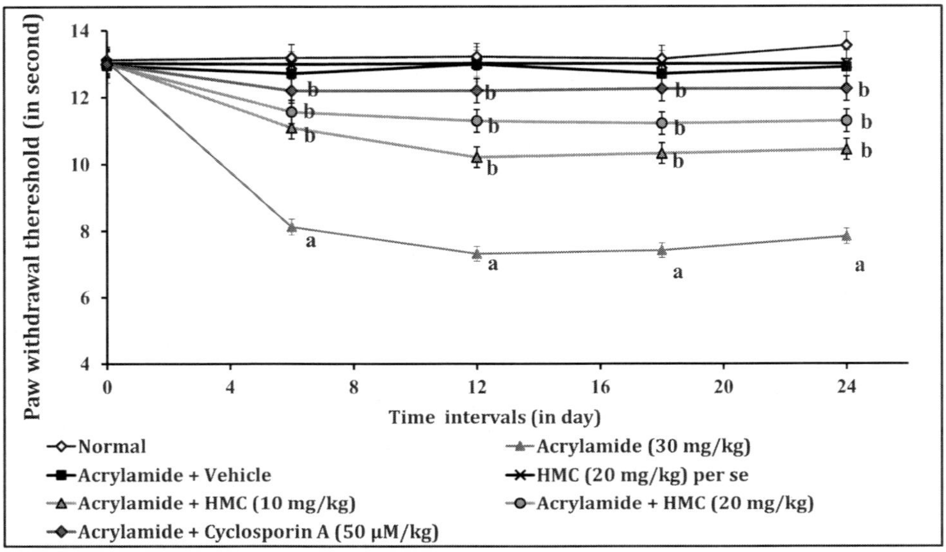

Fig. (2). Effect of HMC on plantar test
HMC, 7-hydroxy-4-methylcoumarin.
Data were expressed as mean ± SD, six animal per group (n=6) were used for the statistical analysis.
[a]$P < 0.05$ *versus* normal control group.
[b]$P < 0.05$ *versus* acrylamide control group.

Effect of HMC on Hot Plate Test

The administration of acrylamide (30 mg/kg) resulted in a significant development of conduction heat hyperalgesia as indicated by a decrease in right hind paw withdrawal threshold after the 6th day of acrylamide intoxication when compared to a normal control group. Administration of HMC (10 and 20 mg/kg) attenuated acrylamide induced decrease in the thermal nociceptive pain threshold in a dose dependent manner. Treatment of cyclosporin A (CsA, 50 μM/kg) also produced similar effects. However, HMC *per se* and vehicle treated group did not show any significant ($P > 0.05$) change in acrylamide induced thermal hyperalgesia (Fig. **3**).

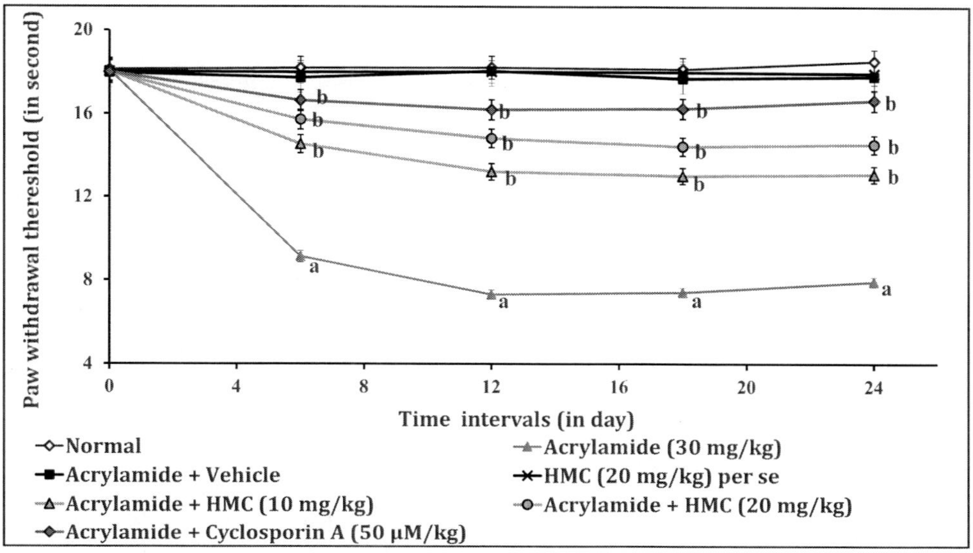

Fig. (3). Effect of HMC on hot plate test.
HMC, 7-hydroxy-4-methylcoumarin.
Data were expressed as mean ± SD, six animal per group (n=6) were used for the statistical analysis.
[a]$P < 0.05$ *versus* normal control group.
[b]$P < 0.05$ *versus* acrylamide control group.

Effect of HMC on Von Frey Hair Test

The administration of acrylamide (30 mg/kg) resulted in a significant development of tactile mechanical allodynia as indicated by a rise in the percentage paw withdrawal response after the 6th day of acrylamide intoxication when compared to a normal control group. Administration of HMC (10 and 20 mg/kg) attenuated acrylamide induced rise in mechanical allodynia response in a dose dependant manner. Treatment of cyclosporin A (CsA, 50 µM/kg) also produced similar effects. However, HMC *per se* and vehicle treated group did not show any significant ($P > 0.05$) change in acrylamide induced mechanical allodynic response (Fig. **4**).

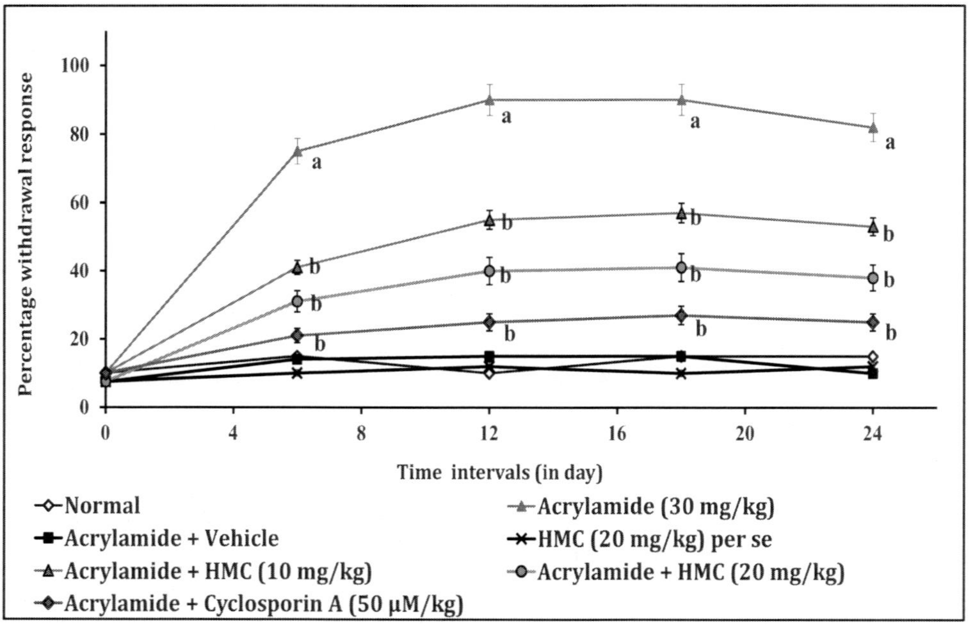

Fig. (4). Effect of HMC on Von Frey Hair test.
HMC, 7-hydroxy-4-methylcoumarin.
Data were expressed as mean ± SD, six animal per group (n=6) were used for the statistical analysis.
[a]$P < 0.05$ *versus* normal control group.
[b]$P < 0.05$ *versus* acrylamide control group.

Effect of HMC on Tail Immersion Test

The administration of acrylamide (30 mg/kg) resulted in a significant development of thermal hyperalgesia as indicated by a decrease in tail withdrawal threshold after the 6th day of acrylamide intoxication when compared to a normal control group. Administration of HMC (10 and 20 mg/kg) attenuated acrylamide induced decrease in tail withdrawal threshold in a dose dependant manner. Treatment of cyclosporin A (CsA, 50 µM/kg) also produced similar effects. However, HMC *per se* and vehicle treated group did not show any significant ($P > 0.05$) change in acrylamide induced thermal hyperalgesia (Fig. **5**).

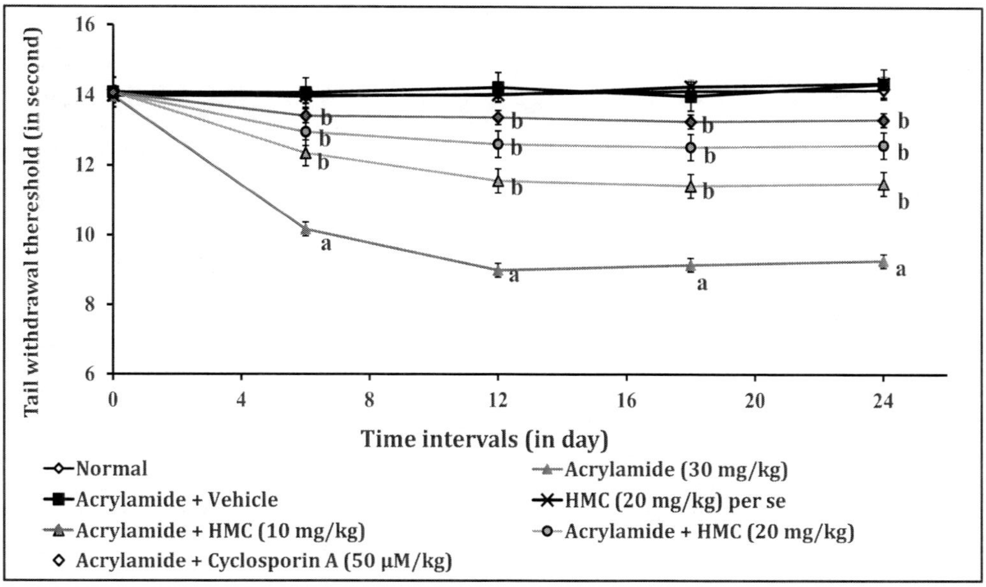

Fig. (5). Effect of HMC on tail immersion test

HMC, 7-hydroxy-4-methylcoumarin.

Data were expressed as mean ± SD, six animal per group (n=6) were used for the statistical analysis.

[a]$P < 0.05$ *versus* normal control group.

[b]$P < 0.05$ *versus* acrylamide control group.

Effect of HMC on Tissue Biomarker Changes

The administration of acrylamide (30 mg/kg) resulted in a significant rise in TBARS, and total calcium levels and decrease in GSH, cytochrome c oxidase activity and ATP content levels after the 24th day of acrylamide intoxication when compared to a normal control group. Administration of HMC (10 and 20 mg/kg) attenuated acrylamide induced biochemical changes mentioned above in a dose dependant manner. Treatment of cyclosporin A (CsA, 50 µM/kg) also produced similar effects. However, HMC *per se* and vehicle treated group did not show any significant ($P > 0.05$) change in above biochemical markers (Tables **1** and **2**).

Table 1. Effect of HMC on acrylamide induced tissue biomarker changes.

Groups	TBARS (nM / mg of protein)	GSH (µM / mg of protein)	Total Calcium (ppm / mg of protein)
Normal	3.21 ± 0.65	73.81 ± 2.37	3.98 ± 1.22
Acrylamide	7.96 ± 0.74 [a]	43.98 ± 2.74 [a]	36.07 ± 1.56 [a]
Acrylamide + Vehicle	8.04 ± 0.72 [a]	42.72 ± 2.68 [a]	34.86 ± 1.94 [a]
HMC (20 mg/kg) *per se*	3.17 ± 0.83	72.96 ± 2.29	3.65 ± 1.71
Acrylamide + HMC (10 mg/kg)	4.82 ± 0.62 [b]	61.38 ± 2.14 [b]	11.87 ± 1.68 [b]
Acrylamide + HMC (20 mg/kg)	4.39 ± 0.89 [b]	64.06 ± 2.35 [b]	7.52 ± 1.84 [b]
Acrylamide + Cyclosporin A (50 µM/kg)	3.73 ± 0.78 [b]	70.83 ± 2.59 [b]	4.52 ± 1.91 [b]

HMC, 7-hydroxy-4-methylcoumarin; TBARS, thiobarbituric reactive substance; GSH, reduced glutathione.
Data were expressed as mean ± SD, six animal per group (n=6) were used for the statistical analysis.
[a]$P < 0.05$ *versus* normal control group.
[b]$P < 0.05$ *versus* acrylamide control group

Table 2. Effect of HMC on acrylamide induced mitochondrial functional changes.

Groups	Cytochrome c oxidase (nM / min / mg of protein)	ATP content (pM / mg of protein)
Normal	0.92 ± 0.01	389.21 ± 3.76
Acrylamide	0.17 ± 0.03 [a]	215.45 ± 5.21
Acrylamide + Vehicle	0.22 ± 0.02 [a]	211.96 ± 4.72 [a]
HMC (20 mg/kg) *per se*	0.91 ± 0.02	383.68 ± 4.58
Acrylamide + HMC (10 mg/kg)	0.52 ± 0.04 [b]	299.05 ± 5.43 [b]
Acrylamide + HMC (20 mg/kg)	0.61 ± 0.03 [b]	347.71 ± 4.36 [b]
Acrylamide + Cyclosporin A (50 µM/kg)	0.84 ± 0.01 [b]	376.92 ± 3.94 [b]

HMC, 7-hydroxy-4-methylcoumarin; ATP, adenosine triphosphate.
Data were expressed as mean ± SD, six animal per group (n=6) were used for the statistical analysis.
[a]$P < 0.05$ *versus* normal control group.
[b]$P < 0.05$ *versus* acrylamide control group.

DISCUSSION

In the present study, administration of HMC attenuated acrylamide (30 mg/kg; *i.p.*) induced nociceptive neuropathic pain appears as an index of thermal and mechanical pain sensation in rat paw and tail regions. In addition, it also ameliorates the acrylamide induced rise in TBARS and total calcium, fall in GSH, cytochrome c oxidase activity and ATP content levels. It indicates that, acrylamide treatment causes the central as well as peripheral neuropathic pain in rats. Whereas, the treatment of HMC ameliorates the neuropathic pain by alteration of neuronal free radical mediators and mitochondrial function markers.

Acrylamide is one of major neurotoxic chemical and it alters the mitochondrial function [25, 63]. Nerve tissue is the highest energy utilizing tissue in the body. Various factors alter the neuronal functions like internal factors, *i.e.,* ischemia, hypoxia, thrombosis, uremia, diabetes, obesity, endocrine abnormality and stress; and external factors, *i.e.,* alcohol drinking, radiation, smoking, surgery, physical and mechanical injury [64 - 66]. In pathological conditions, nerve undergoes the neurodegeneration due to various physiological processes like free radical generation; accumulation of calcium and calcium binding proteins (*i.e.,* calcineurin, calmodulin and calpain); over expression of pro-apoptotic (*i.e.,* Bax, Bak, BAD and Bok), pro-inflammatory (*i.e.,* TNF-α and interleukin-1) proteins; and various cytokines and chemokines [67 - 69]. The above all mechanisms are responsible in acrylamide induced neurodegeneration and cause the neuropathic pain. This molecular mechanism is closely related to mitochondria, because, it is an energy producing organelle and also modulates the free radical formation and calcium homeostasis function in the intracellular environments [69 - 71]. The abnormality of cytosolic calcium and free radicals contributes to the progress of mitochondrial dysfunction in the nervous system [72, 73].

Wallerian degeneration is one of the key events of the neurodegeneration in the peripheral nervous system and it is also known to produce the neuropathic pain *via* activation of m-calpain protein [74, 75]. In addition, cytosolic calcium accumulation contributes in neuronal oxidative stress, lipid peroxidation and opening of mitochondrial permeability transition pore (MPTP) which is also identified in the pathogenesis of neuropathic pain [76 - 79].

Reduced glutathione is an endogenous anti-oxidant molecule and it also contributes in nutrient metabolism and regulation of cellular survival as well as functional events [54, 80]. The deficiency of GSH contributes in the oxidative stress during various disorders, *i.e.,* hepatic, renal failure, cardiac failure,

Alzheimer's disease, Parkinson disease and neuropathic pain [81 - 84]. Furthermore, glutathione molecule also possesses the detoxifying property against neurotoxic metabolite of acrylamide (*i.e.,* glycidamide (2, 3-epoxy-1-propanamide) by glutathione conjugation process [85, 86].

Mitochondrial dysfunction is the key event in the progress of neurodegeneration and neuropathic pain. Acrylamide known to cause the mitochondrial dysfunction in the nervous system *via* opening of MPTP [46, 47], which enhances the free radical generation and expression of various proapoptotic proteins [87]. In addition, opening of MPTP is known to release the free radical, cytochrome c and alters the mitochondrial membrane potential [88, 89]. The cyclosporine A is known to inhibit the MPTP opening and regulates the cellular function in the nervous system [45, 90].

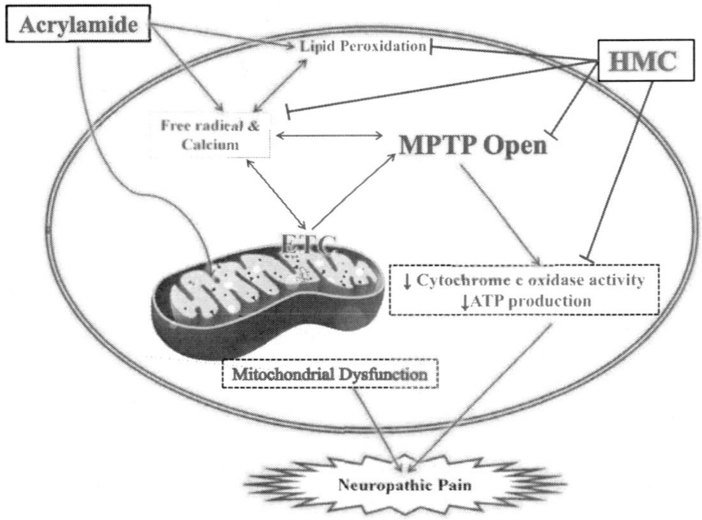

Fig. (6). The possible molecular mechanism of HMC in the ameliorative effect of acrylamide induced neuropathic pain. HMC attenuates the neuropathic pain symptoms due to its anti-oxidative, anti-lipidperoxidative and calcium modulatory actions. In addition, it also regulates the mitochondrial function by reducing the cytochrome c oxidase activity and improvement of ATP production *via* inhibition of MPTP opening. ETC, electron transport chain; and HMC, 7-hydroxy-4-methylcoumarin.

Coumarin has been reported to prevent the various ailments, *i.e.,* anti-psychotic [37], anti-thrombotic [38] and anti-diabetic [39] and improvement of learning and memory function [42]. The present study endorses the view point that, coumarin possesses the anti-oxidant and anti-inflammatory actions by rising of GSH and reducing the TBARS levels [91, 92]. Coumarin derivative is also known to prevent the calcium induced neuronal death *via* raising the expression of hippocalcin [93]. It also produces the potential action on mitochondrial functional regulation [44]. In addition, cyclosporine A is believed to be neuroprotective *via* regulation of mitochondrial function by inhibition of MPTP opening and release of cytochrome c [45]. Similar results have been observed in the present study. The molecular hypothesis of this research work has been illustrated in Fig. (**6**).

The pretreatment of HMC attenuates the acrylamide induced neuropathic pain along with various biochemical alterations, *i.e.,* TBARS, GSH, total calcium, cytochrome c oxidase and ATP contents.

CONCLUSION

The HMC possesses the ameliorative effect in acrylamide induced neuropathic pain in rats. It may be due to its potential blocking actions of intracellular calcium ion accumulation, free radical generation, lipid peroxidation and mitochondrial dysfunction. More extensive studies are needed to explore full therapeutic potential of HMC against various neurotoxic chemicals along with a précised molecular mechanism in the management of neuropathic pain disorder.

CONFLICT OF INTEREST

The authors confirm that they have no conflict of interest to declare for this publication.

ACKNOWLEDGEMENTS

The authors are thankful to all faculty members of Akal College of Pharmacy & Technical Education, Mastuana Sahib, Sangrur-148002, Punjab, India for their valuable suggestions and support to carry out this research work.

REFERENCES

[1] O'Connor AB, Dworkin RH. Treatment of neuropathic pain: an overview of recent guidelines. Am J Med 2009; 122(10) (Suppl.): S22-32.

[http://dx.doi.org/10.1016/j.amjmed.2009.04.007] [PMID: 19801049]

[2] Woolf CJ, Mannion RJ. Neuropathic pain: aetiology, symptoms, mechanisms, and management. Lancet 1999; 353(9168): 1959-64.
[http://dx.doi.org/10.1016/S0140-6736(99)01307-0] [PMID: 10371588]

[3] Dworkin RH, O'Connor AB, Audette J, *et al.* Recommendations for the pharmacological management of neuropathic pain: an overview and literature update. Mayo Clin Proc 2010; 85(3) (Suppl.): S3-S14.
[http://dx.doi.org/10.4065/mcp.2009.0649] [PMID: 20194146]

[4] Lee J, Nandi P. Improving the management of neuropathic pain. Practitioner 2010; 254(1731): 27-30, 3.
[PMID: 20812611]

[5] Hammersla M, Kapustin JF. Peripheral neuropathy: evidence-based treatment of a complex disorder. Nurse Pract 2012; 37(5): 32-9.
[http://dx.doi.org/10.1097/01.NPR.0000413482.44379.ff] [PMID: 22460540]

[6] Jaggi AS, Singh N. Therapeutic targets for the management of peripheral nerve injury-induced neuropathic pain. CNS Neurol Disord Drug Targets 2011; 10(5): 589-609.
[http://dx.doi.org/10.2174/187152711796235041] [PMID: 21631400]

[7] Jaggi AS, Jain V, Singh N. Animal models of neuropathic pain. Fundam Clin Pharmacol 2011; 25(1): 1-28.
[http://dx.doi.org/10.1111/j.1472-8206.2009.00801.x] [PMID: 20030738]

[8] Ren JL, Peng F, Sun RC. Preparation and characterization of hemicellulosic derivatives containing carbamoylethyl and carboxyethyl groups. Carbohydr Res 2008; 343(16): 2776-82.
[http://dx.doi.org/10.1016/j.carres.2008.05.019] [PMID: 18561904]

[9] Wang CC, Lee CM. Denitrification with acrylamide by pure culture of bacteria isolated from acrylonitrile-butadiene-styrene resin manufactured wastewater treatment system. Chemosphere 2001; 44(5): 1047-53.
[http://dx.doi.org/10.1016/S0045-6535(00)00503-8] [PMID: 11513390]

[10] Blancher C, Cormick RM. Sodium dodecyl sulphate-polyacrylamide denaturing gel electrophoresis and Western blotting techniques. Methods Mol Biol 2012; 878: 89-110.
[http://dx.doi.org/10.1007/978-1-61779-854-2_6] [PMID: 22674128]

[11] Bonacucina G, Cespi M, Palmieri GF. Characterization and stability of emulsion gels based on acrylamide/sodium acryloyldimethyl taurate copolymer. AAPS PharmSciTech 2009; 10(2): 368-75.
[http://dx.doi.org/10.1208/s12249-009-9218-1] [PMID: 19340587]

[12] Boroushaki MT, Nikkhah E, Kazemi A, Oskooei M, Raters M. Determination of acrylamide level in popular Iranian brands of potato and corn products. Food Chem Toxicol 2010; 48(10): 2581-4.
[http://dx.doi.org/10.1016/j.fct.2010.06.011] [PMID: 20600544]

[13] Lofstedt RE. Science communication and the Swedish acrylamide "alarm". J Health Commun 2003; 8(5): 407-32.
[http://dx.doi.org/10.1080/713852123] [PMID: 14530144]

[14] Xu XM, He HL, Zhu Y, *et al.* Simultaneous determination of 3-monochloropropane-1,2-diol and acrylamide in food by gas chromatography-triple quadrupole mass spectrometry with coupled column

separation. Anal Chim Acta 2013; 760: 93-9.
[http://dx.doi.org/10.1016/j.aca.2012.11.036] [PMID: 23265738]

[15] Mucci LA, Sandin S, Bälter K, Adami HO, Magnusson C, Weiderpass E. Acrylamide intake and breast cancer risk in Swedish women. JAMA 2005; 293(11): 1326-7.
[PMID: 15769965]

[16] Chen YH, Xia EQ, Xu XR, *et al.* Evaluation of acrylamide in food from China by a LC/MS/MS method. Int J Environ Res Public Health 2012; 9(11): 4150-8.
[http://dx.doi.org/10.3390/ijerph9114150] [PMID: 23202837]

[17] Mottram DS, Wedzicha BL, Dodson AT. Acrylamide is formed in the Maillard reaction. Nature 2002; 419(6906): 448-9.
[http://dx.doi.org/10.1038/419448a] [PMID: 12368844]

[18] Adewale OO, Brimson JM, Odunola OA, *et al.* The Potential for Plant Derivatives against Acrylamide Neurotoxicity. Phytother Res 2015; 29(7): 978-85.
[http://dx.doi.org/10.1002/ptr.5353] [PMID: 25886076]

[19] Jiang H, Xiang Y, Hu X, Cai H. Acrylamide inhibits nerve sprouting induced by botulinum toxin type A. Neural Regen Res 2014; 9(16): 1525-31.
[http://dx.doi.org/10.4103/1673-5374.139479] [PMID: 25317170]

[20] Ahmed HH, Elmegeed GA, el-Sayed SM, Abd-Elhalim MM, Shousha WG, Shafic RW. Potent neuroprotective role of novel melatonin derivatives for management of central neuropathy induced by acrylamide in rats. Eur J Med Chem 2010; 45(11): 5452-9.
[http://dx.doi.org/10.1016/j.ejmech.2010.09.017] [PMID: 20870314]

[21] Comblath DR. Neuropathy in grout workers. Scand J Work Environ Health 2004; 30(3): 253-4.
[http://dx.doi.org/10.5271/sjweh.787] [PMID: 15250655]

[22] Lehning EJ, Balaban CD, Ross JF, Reid MA, LoPachin RM. Acrylamide neuropathy. I. Spatiotemporal characteristics of nerve cell damage in rat cerebellum. Neurotoxicology 2002; 23(3): 397-414.
[http://dx.doi.org/10.1016/S0161-813X(02)00083-9] [PMID: 12387366]

[23] Ling B, Authier N, Balayssac D, Eschalier A, Coudore F. Assessment of nociception in acrylamide-induced neuropathy in rats. Pain 2005; 119(1-3): 104-12.
[http://dx.doi.org/10.1016/j.pain.2005.09.021] [PMID: 16298070]

[24] Raygude KS, Kandhare AD, Ghosh P, Ghule AE, Bodhankar SL. Evaluation of ameliorative effect of quercetin in experimental model of alcoholic neuropathy in rats. Inflammopharmacology 2012; 20(6): 331-41.
[http://dx.doi.org/10.1007/s10787-012-0122-z] [PMID: 22349996]

[25] Prasad SN, Muralidhara . Neuroprotective effect of geraniol and curcumin in an acrylamide model of neurotoxicity in Drosophila melanogaster: relevance to neuropathy. J Insect Physiol 2014; 60: 7-16.
[http://dx.doi.org/10.1016/j.jinsphys.2013.10.003] [PMID: 24231732]

[26] Tamaddonfard E, Farshid AA, Maroufi S, *et al.* Effects of safranal, a constituent of saffron, and vitamin E on nerve functions and histopathology following crush injury of sciatic nerve in rats. Phytomedicine 2014; 21(5): 717-23.

[http://dx.doi.org/10.1016/j.phymed.2013.10.031] [PMID: 24315349]

[27] Liu M, Liao K, Yu C, *et al.* Puerarin alleviates neuropathic pain by inhibiting neuroinflammation in spinal cord 2014. [http://dx.doi.org/10.1155/2014/485927]

[28] Amin B, Taheri MM, Hosseinzadeh H. Effects of intraperitoneal thymoquinone on chronic neuropathic pain in rats. Planta Med 2014; 80(15): 1269-77. [http://dx.doi.org/10.1055/s-0034-1383062] [PMID: 25272235]

[29] Chipiti T, Ibrahim MA, Koorbanally NA, Islam MS. *In vitro* antioxidant activities of leaf and root extracts of *Albizia antunesiana* harms. Acta Pol Pharm 2013; 70(6): 1035-43. [PMID: 24383327]

[30] Bajerová P, Adam M, Bajer T, Ventura K. Comparison of various techniques for the extraction and determination of antioxidants in plants. J Sep Sci 2014; 37(7): 835-44. [http://dx.doi.org/10.1002/jssc.201301139] [PMID: 24470390]

[31] Nurul Islam M, Jung HA, Sohn HS, Kim HM, Choi JS. Potent α-glucosidase and protein tyrosine phosphatase 1B inhibitors from Artemisia capillaris. Arch Pharm Res 2013; 36(5): 542-52. [http://dx.doi.org/10.1007/s12272-013-0069-7] [PMID: 23435948]

[32] Ezzat SM, Abdallah HM, Fawzy GA, El-Maraghy SA. Hepatoprotective constituents of *Torilis radiata Moench* (*Apiaceae*). Nat Prod Res 2012; 26(3): 282-5. [http://dx.doi.org/10.1080/14786419.2011.587422] [PMID: 21867456]

[33] van Schie RM, Babajeff AM, Schalekamp T, *et al.* An evaluation of gene-gene interaction between the CYP2C9 and VKORC1 genotypes affecting the anticoagulant effect of phenprocoumon and acenocoumarol. J Thromb Haemost 2012; 10(5): 767-72. [http://dx.doi.org/10.1111/j.1538-7836.2012.04694.x] [PMID: 22409277]

[34] Basanagouda M, Shivashankar K, Kulkarni MV, *et al.* Synthesis and antimicrobial studies on novel sulfonamides containing 4-azidomethyl coumarin. Eur J Med Chem 2010; 45(3): 1151-7. [http://dx.doi.org/10.1016/j.ejmech.2009.12.022] [PMID: 20047777]

[35] Zhang L, Jiang G, Yao F, *et al.* Growth inhibition and apoptosis induced by osthole, a natural coumarin, in hepatocellular carcinoma. PLoS One 2012; 7(5): e37865. [http://dx.doi.org/10.1371/journal.pone.0037865] [PMID: 22662241]

[36] Witaicenis A, Luchini AC, Hiruma-Lima CA, *et al.* Suppression of TNBS-induced colitis in rats by 4-methylesculetin, a natural coumarin: comparison with prednisolone and sulphasalazine. Chem Biol Interact 2012; 195(1): 76-85. [http://dx.doi.org/10.1016/j.cbi.2011.11.004] [PMID: 22119283]

[37] Chen Y, Wang S, Xu X, *et al.* Synthesis and biological investigation of coumarin piperazine (piperidine) derivatives as potential multireceptor atypical antipsychotics. J Med Chem 2013; 56(11): 4671-90. [http://dx.doi.org/10.1021/jm400408r] [PMID: 23675993]

[38] Jain M, Surin WR, Misra A, *et al.* Antithrombotic activity of a newly synthesized coumarin derivative 3-(5-hydroxy-2,2-dimethyl-chroman-6-yl)-N-2-[3-(5-hydroxy-2,2-dimet-yl-chroman-6-yl)-propionylamino]-ethyl-propionamide. Chem Biol Drug Des 2013; 81(4): 499-508.

[http://dx.doi.org/10.1111/cbdd.12000] [PMID: 23534412]

[39] Han J, Sun L, Huang X, *et al.* Novel coumarin modified GLP-1 derivatives with enhanced plasma stability and prolonged *in vivo* glucose-lowering ability. Br J Pharmacol 2014; 171(23): 5252-64. [http://dx.doi.org/10.1111/bph.12843] [PMID: 25039358]

[40] Miri R, Nejati M, Saso L, *et al.* Structure-activity relationship studies of 4-methylcoumarin derivatives as anticancer agents. Pharm Biol 2015; 1-6. [PMID: 26017566]

[41] El-Haggar R, Al-Wabli RI. Anti-inflammatory screening and molecular modeling of some novel coumarin derivatives. Molecules 2015; 20(4): 5374-91. [http://dx.doi.org/10.3390/molecules20045374] [PMID: 25822078]

[42] Zuo W, Zhang W, Han N, Chen NH. Compound IMM-H004, a novel coumarin derivative, protects against CA_1 cell loss and spatial learning impairments resulting from transient global ischemia. CNS Neurosci Ther 2015; 21(3): 280-8. [http://dx.doi.org/10.1111/cns.12364] [PMID: 25601434]

[43] Jing WH, Song YL, Yan R, Wang YT. Identification of cytochrome P450 isoenzymes involved in metabolism of (+)-praeruptorin A, a calcium channel blocker, by human liver microsomes using ultra high-performance liquid chromatography coupled with tandem mass spectrometry. J Pharm Biomed Anal 2013; 77: 175-88. [http://dx.doi.org/10.1016/j.jpba.2013.01.023] [PMID: 23434495]

[44] Bronikowska J, Szliszka E, Jaworska D, Czuba ZP, Krol W. The coumarin psoralidin enhances anticancer effect of tumor necrosis factor-related apoptosis-inducing ligand (TRAIL). Molecules 2012; 17(6): 6449-64. [http://dx.doi.org/10.3390/molecules17066449] [PMID: 22643355]

[45] Kim WS, Park JY, Kim TK, Baik SW. The changes of mitochondrial cytochrome c and GABAergic neuron in neuropathic pain model. Korean J Anesthesiol 2012; 62(4): 365-70. [http://dx.doi.org/10.4097/kjae.2012.62.4.365] [PMID: 22558504]

[46] Liu Z, Song G, Zou C, *et al.* Acrylamide induces mitochondrial dysfunction and apoptosis in BV-2 microglial cells. Free Radic Biol Med 2015; 84: 42-53. [http://dx.doi.org/10.1016/j.freeradbiomed.2015.03.013] [PMID: 25817051]

[47] Fancelli D, Abate A, Amici R, *et al.* Cinnamic anilides as new mitochondrial permeability transition pore inhibitors endowed with ischemia-reperfusion injury protective effect *in vivo.* J Med Chem 2014; 57(12): 5333-47. [http://dx.doi.org/10.1021/jm500547c] [PMID: 24918261]

[48] Gold BG, Voda J, Yu X, Gordon H. The immunosuppressant FK506 elicits a neuronal heat shock response and protects against acrylamide neuropathy. Exp Neurol 2004; 187(1): 160-70. [http://dx.doi.org/10.1016/j.expneurol.2004.01.005] [PMID: 15081597]

[49] Choi Y, Yoon YW, Na HS, Kim SH, Chung JM. Behavioral signs of ongoing pain and cold allodynia in a rat model of neuropathic pain. Pain 1994; 59(3): 369-76. [http://dx.doi.org/10.1016/0304-3959(94)90023-X] [PMID: 7708411]

[50] Hargreaves K, Dubner R, Brown F, Flores C, Joris J. A new and sensitive method for measuring

thermal nociception in cutaneous hyperalgesia. Pain 1988; 32(1): 77-88.
[http://dx.doi.org/10.1016/0304-3959(88)90026-7] [PMID: 3340425]

[51] Eddy NB, Touchberry CF, Lieberman JE. Synthetic analgesics; methadone isomers and derivatives. J Pharmacol Exp Ther 1950; 98(2): 121-37.
[PMID: 15422505]

[52] Chaplan SR, Bach FW, Pogrel JW, Chung JM, Yaksh TL. Quantitative assessment of tactile allodynia in the rat paw. J Neurosci Methods 1994; 53(1): 55-63.
[http://dx.doi.org/10.1016/0165-0270(94)90144-9] [PMID: 7990513]

[53] Necker R, Hellon RF. Noxious thermal input from the rat tail: modulation by descending inhibitory influences. Pain 1978; 4(3): 231-42.
[PMID: 634623]

[54] Muthuraman A, Diwan V, Jaggi AS, Singh N, Singh D. Ameliorative effects of *Ocimum sanctum* in sciatic nerve transection-induced neuropathy in rats. J Ethnopharmacol 2008; 120(1): 56-62.
[http://dx.doi.org/10.1016/j.jep.2008.07.049] [PMID: 18762236]

[55] Lowry OH, Rosebrough NJ, Farr AL, Randall RJ. Protein measurement with the Folin phenol reagent. J Biol Chem 1951; 193(1): 265-75.
[PMID: 14907713]

[56] Niehaus WG Jr, Samuelsson B. Formation of malonaldehyde from phospholipid arachidonate during microsomal lipid peroxidation. Eur J Biochem 1968; 6(1): 126-30.
[http://dx.doi.org/10.1111/j.1432-1033.1968.tb00428.x] [PMID: 4387188]

[57] Beutler E, Duron O, Kelly BM. Improved method for the determination of blood glutathione. J Lab Clin Med 1963; 61: 882-8.
[PMID: 13967893]

[58] Severinghaus JW, Ferrebee JW. Calcium determination by flame photometry; methods for serum, urine, and other fluids. J Biol Chem 1950; 187(2): 621-30.
[PMID: 14803444]

[59] Viader A, Golden JP, Baloh RH, Schmidt RE, Hunter DA, Milbrandt J. Schwann cell mitochondrial metabolism supports long-term axonal survival and peripheral nerve function. J Neurosci 2011; 31(28): 10128-40.
[http://dx.doi.org/10.1523/JNEUROSCI.0884-11.2011] [PMID: 21752989]

[60] Frezza C, Cipolat S, Scorrano L. Organelle isolation: functional mitochondria from mouse liver, muscle and cultured fibroblasts. Nat Protoc 2007; 2(2): 287-95.
[http://dx.doi.org/10.1038/nprot.2006.478] [PMID: 17406588]

[61] Rustin P, Chretien D, Bourgeron T, *et al.* Biochemical and molecular investigations in respiratory chain deficiencies. Clin Chim Acta 1994; 228(1): 35-51.
[http://dx.doi.org/10.1016/0009-8981(94)90055-8] [PMID: 7955428]

[62] Ally A, Park G. Rapid determination of creatine, phosphocreatine, purine bases and nucleotides (ATP, ADP, AMP, GTP, GDP) in heart biopsies by gradient ion-pair reversed-phase liquid chromatography. J Chromatogr A 1992; 575(1): 19-27.
[http://dx.doi.org/10.1016/0378-4347(92)80499-G] [PMID: 1517298]

[63] Lehning EJ, Persaud A, Dyer KR, Jortner BS, LoPachin RM. Biochemical and morphologic characterization of acrylamide peripheral neuropathy. Toxicol Appl Pharmacol 1998; 151(2): 211-21. [http://dx.doi.org/10.1006/taap.1998.8464] [PMID: 9707497]

[64] Nguyen DV, Shaw LC, Grant MB. Inflammation in the pathogenesis of microvascular complications in diabetes. Front Endocrinol (Lausanne) 2012; 3: 170. [http://dx.doi.org/10.3389/fendo.2012.00170] [PMID: 23267348]

[65] Tweed JO, Hsia SH, Lutfy K, Friedman TC. The endocrine effects of nicotine and cigarette smoke. Trends Endocrinol Metab 2012; 23(7): 334-42. [http://dx.doi.org/10.1016/j.tem.2012.03.006] [PMID: 22561025]

[66] Starcke K, van Holst RJ, van den Brink W, Veltman DJ, Goudriaan AE. Physiological and endocrine reactions to psychosocial stress in alcohol use disorders: duration of abstinence matters. Alcohol Clin Exp Res 2013; 37(8): 1343-50. [http://dx.doi.org/10.1111/acer.12103] [PMID: 23488992]

[67] Martin LJ. Mitochondrial and cell death mechanisms in neurodegenerative diseases. Pharmaceuticals (Basel) 2010; 3(4): 839-915. [http://dx.doi.org/10.3390/ph3040839] [PMID: 21258649]

[68] Natarajan SK, Becker DF. Role of apoptosis-inducing factor, proline dehydrogenase, and NADPH oxidase in apoptosis and oxidative stress 2012.

[69] Yakovlev AG, Faden AI. Mechanisms of neural cell death: implications for development of neuroprotective treatment strategies. NeuroRx 2004; 1(1): 5-16. [http://dx.doi.org/10.1602/neurorx.1.1.5] [PMID: 15717003]

[70] Roh SE, Woo JA, Lakshmana MK, *et al.* Mitochondrial dysfunction and calcium deregulation by the RanBP9-cofilin pathway. FASEB J 2013; 27(12): 4776-89. [http://dx.doi.org/10.1096/fj.13-234765] [PMID: 23982146]

[71] Mustafa AG, Singh IN, Wang J, Carrico KM, Hall ED. Mitochondrial protection after traumatic brain injury by scavenging lipid peroxyl radicals. J Neurochem 2010; 114(1): 271-80. [PMID: 20403083]

[72] Martinc B, Grabnar I, Vovk T. The role of reactive species in epileptogenesis and influence of antiepileptic drug therapy on oxidative stress. Curr Neuropharmacol 2012; 10(4): 328-43. [http://dx.doi.org/10.2174/1570159X11209040328] [PMID: 23730257]

[73] Kumar H, Lim HW, More SV, *et al.* The role of free radicals in the aging brain and Parkinson's Disease: convergence and parallelism. Int J Mol Sci 2012; 13(8): 10478-504. [http://dx.doi.org/10.3390/ijms130810478] [PMID: 22949875]

[74] Glass JD, Culver DG, Levey AI, Nash NR. Very early activation of m-calpain in peripheral nerve during Wallerian degeneration. J Neurol Sci 2002; 196(1-2): 9-20. [http://dx.doi.org/10.1016/S0022-510X(02)00013-8] [PMID: 11959150]

[75] Muthuraman A, Singh N. Neuroprotective effect of saponin rich extract of *Acorus calamus* L. in rat model of chronic constriction injury (CCI) of sciatic nerve-induced neuropathic pain. J Ethnopharmacol 2012; 142(3): 723-31. [http://dx.doi.org/10.1016/j.jep.2012.05.049] [PMID: 22706151]

[76] Maciel EN, Vercesi AE, Castilho RF. Oxidative stress in Ca(2+)-induced membrane permeability transition in brain mitochondria. J Neurochem 2001; 79(6): 1237-45. [http://dx.doi.org/10.1046/j.1471-4159.2001.00670.x] [PMID: 11752064]

[77] Muthuraman A, Singh N. Attenuating effect of *Acorus calamus* extract in chronic constriction injury induced neuropathic pain in rats: an evidence of anti-oxidative, anti-inflammatory, neuroprotective and calcium inhibitory effects. BMC Complement Altern Med 2011; 11: 24. [http://dx.doi.org/10.1186/1472-6882-11-24] [PMID: 21426568]

[78] Muthuraman A, Singh N, Jaggi AS. Protective effect of *Acorus calamus* L. in rat model of vincristine induced painful neuropathy: an evidence of anti-inflammatory and anti-oxidative activity. Food Chem Toxicol 2011; 49(10): 2557-63. [http://dx.doi.org/10.1016/j.fct.2011.06.069] [PMID: 21756962]

[79] Teepker M, Anthes N, Fischer S, Krieg JC, Vedder H. Effects of oxidative challenge and calcium on ATP-levels in neuronal cells. Neurotoxicology 2007; 28(1): 19-26. [http://dx.doi.org/10.1016/j.neuro.2006.06.001] [PMID: 16870261]

[80] Muthuraman A, Ramesh M, Sood S. Development of animal model for vasculatic neuropathy: Induction by ischemic-reperfusion in the rat femoral artery. J Neurosci Methods 2010; 186(2): 215-21. [http://dx.doi.org/10.1016/j.jneumeth.2009.12.004] [PMID: 20026113]

[81] Gulati P, Muthuraman A, Jaggi AS, Singh N. Neuroprotective effect of gadolinium: a stretch-activated calcium channel blocker in mouse model of ischemia-reperfusion injury. Naunyn Schmiedebergs Arch Pharmacol 2013; 386(3): 255-64. [http://dx.doi.org/10.1007/s00210-012-0819-y] [PMID: 23229582]

[82] Muthuraman A, Jaggi AS, Singh N, Singh D. Ameliorative effects of amiloride and pralidoxime in chronic constriction injury and vincristine induced painful neuropathy in rats. Eur J Pharmacol 2008; 587(1-3): 104-11. [http://dx.doi.org/10.1016/j.ejphar.2008.03.042] [PMID: 18486127]

[83] Muthuraman A, Sood S. Pharmacological evaluation of tacrolimus (FK-506) on ischemia reperfusion induced vasculatic neuropathic pain in rats. J Brachial Plex Peripher Nerve Inj 2010; 5: 13. [PMID: 20529260]

[84] Pinnen F, Sozio P, Cacciatore I, *et al.* Ibuprofen and glutathione conjugate as a potential therapeutic agent for treating Alzheimer's disease. Arch Pharm (Weinheim) 2011; 344(3): 139-48. [http://dx.doi.org/10.1002/ardp.201000209] [PMID: 21384412]

[85] Annola K, Karttunen V, Keski-Rahkonen P, *et al.* Transplacental transfer of acrylamide and glycidamide are comparable to that of antipyrine in perfused human placenta. Toxicol Lett 2008; 182(1-3): 50-6. [http://dx.doi.org/10.1016/j.toxlet.2008.08.006] [PMID: 18790027]

[86] Pernice R, Hauder J, Koehler P, Vitaglione P, Fogliano V, Somoza V. Effect of sulforaphane on glutathione-adduct formation and on glutathione_S_transferase-dependent detoxification of acrylamide in Caco-2 cells. Mol Nutr Food Res 2009; 53(12): 1540-50. [http://dx.doi.org/10.1002/mnfr.200900447] [PMID: 19904761]

[87] King AL, Swain TM, Dickinson DA, Lesort MJ, Bailey SM. Chronic ethanol consumption enhances

sensitivity to Ca(2+)-mediated opening of the mitochondrial permeability transition pore and increases cyclophilin D in liver. Am J Physiol Gastrointest Liver Physiol 2010; 299(4): G954-66. [http://dx.doi.org/10.1152/ajpgi.00246.2010] [PMID: 20651005]

[88] Marchi S, Giorgi C, Suski JM, *et al.* itochondria-ros crosstalk in the control of cell death and aging. M J Signal Transduct 2012; 2012: 329635.

[89] Gautier CA, Giaime E, Caballero E, *et al.* Regulation of mitochondrial permeability transition pore by PINK1. Mol Neurodegener 2012; 7: 22. [http://dx.doi.org/10.1186/1750-1326-7-22] [PMID: 22630785]

[90] Kim SY, Shim MS, Kim KY, Weinreb RN, Wheeler LA, Ju WK. Inhibition of cyclophilin D by cyclosporin A promotes retinal ganglion cell survival by preventing mitochondrial alteration in ischemic injury. Cell Death Dis 2014; 5: e1105. [http://dx.doi.org/10.1038/cddis.2014.80] [PMID: 24603333]

[91] Arora RK, Kaur N, Bansal Y, Bansal G. Novel coumarin-benzimidazole derivatives as antioxidants and safer anti-inflammatory agents. Acta Pharm Sin B 2014; 4(5): 368-75. [http://dx.doi.org/10.1016/j.apsb.2014.07.001] [PMID: 26579406]

[92] Witaicenis A, Seito LN, da Silveira Chagas A, *et al.* Antioxidant and intestinal anti-inflammatory effects of plant-derived coumarin derivatives. Phytomedicine 2014; 21(3): 240-6. [http://dx.doi.org/10.1016/j.phymed.2013.09.001] [PMID: 24176844]

[93] Jin X, Wang Y, Li X, *et al.* 7,8-Dihydroxy-4-methylcoumarin provides neuroprotection by increasing hippocalcin expression. Neurotox Res 2015; 27(3): 268-74. [http://dx.doi.org/10.1007/s12640-014-9507-7] [PMID: 25752619]

SUBJECT INDEX

A

Puneetpal Singh (Ed.)

B

C

F

G

H

I

K

L

O

P

R

U

V

Made in United States
North Haven, CT
04 November 2026

21727463R00122